ARE YOU AN OVERWEIGHT PERSON WHO LOVES FOOD?

This book tells you how to change your weight without changing your habits. It isn't going to try to "reform" you. You can eat, sin and still get thin. It gives you tangible, tested tools—shopping lists, brand names, menus and 1027 delicious recipes—for de-calorizing your family's favorite foods.

STOP DIETING!
START LOSING!
by
Ruth West

Stop
Dieting!
Start
Losing!

Ruth West

BANTAM BOOKS · TORONTO · NEW YORK · LONDON

STOP DIETING! START LOSING!

*A Bantam Book / published by arrangement with
E. P. Dutton & Company, Inc.*

PRINTING HISTORY

*Dutton edition published January 1956
6 printings through August 1957*

One chapter, "Drink Beer and Lose Weight," appeared in
ARGOSY *Magazine April 1954, © 1954*

*Bantam edition / April 1957
13 printings through May 1970
Revised Bantam edition / May 1977*

ISBN 0–553–07242–0

Published simultaneously in the United States and Canada

*Bantam Books are published by Bantam Books, Inc. Its trade-
mark, consisting of the words "Bantam Books" and the por-
trayal of a bantam, is registered in the United States Patent
Office and in other countries. Marca Registrada. Bantam
Books, Inc., 666 Fifth Avenue, New York, New York 10019.*

PRINTED IN THE UNITED STATES OF AMERICA

Contents

Introduction   ix

1   Like Mother Used to Make—Minus Calories!   1

2   How to Modernize Your Recipes   4

3   Six Twentieth-Century Master Recipes   13
    Cream sauce, muffins,
    jiffy waffles, hollandaise for
    moderns, quick-foolproof pastry
    and basic cake and cookie mixes

4   The New Phantom Foods   33

5   Low-Protein Diet or High—Which?   48

6   The Sex-Appeal Sixteen   50

7   Eat Your Milk   56

8   America's Favorte Recipes—De-Calorized   62
    Drinks, canapés, favorite first
    courses, main dishes, vegetables
    and salads, sauces and salad
    dressings and dessert favorites

9   Make Your Kitchen Diet for You   117

10   Fooling Those Alcohol Calories   135

11   How Beer Can Help You Lose Weight   140

12   How Your Husband Can Lose Weight
Without Dieting   145

13 How to Help Yourself Lose Weight   158

Quick Calorie Counter   170

Index   185

Introduction

You've tried dieting. It worked—temporarily, perhaps. At any rate you would still like to lose weight.

Why are we overweight? Because it runs in our families? Because of glandular disorders? Fewer than one-half of one per cent of the people who are overweight can blame it on glandular disorders. The average practitioner is untrained to cope if you confide that your overweight relates to frustration or feelings of insecurity in your life. Psychoanalysts will agree that you have a point, but even if you can afford years of expensive psychotherapy, you may still have trouble keeping your weight down. Among themselves analysts agree to a low success rate here.

What can be done about it?

You can go on a wonder diet. There's a new one every six months. Well, they can lift you out of an over-eating rut. If six to nine pounds is all you want to lose, they may work but—as you know by now—*only temporarily*. The trouble with wonder diets is that while you go through your starvation trial you must withdraw from the world like an anchorite. And, the day you stop the diet routine you begin to gain almost as fast as you lost. That is because to date nobody has told you how to eat all the rich dishes you love—and *still* lose. (And I mean rich *desserts* too!)

You can go on a "sensible" diet. Sensible diets are still very big. "I just cut out desserts, that's all. You know, overweight is just a matter of eating too many sweets with most people." *People who can give up sweets that easily never cared much about them any-*

how. This kind of person, however, often has a weakness for salty, fatty things like salted nuts, and potato chips, all equally loaded with calories.

Recently THE "JUST EAT LESS" solution has been offered under a variety of attractive disguises. There's the gourmet approach, the self-psychoanalytical approach, the "eat everything" approach. But when you get past the beautiful *theory* and into the everyday practice of these preachments you find that they all boil down to either doll-sized portions or A LONG LIST OF TABOO FOODS. In other words, it's the same old prescription: eat less.

If this system worked for most people, very few of us would be overweight. Unfortunately, it only works for a very few because it treats overweight as if it were A SIMPLE PHYSIOLOGICAL PROBLEM. And it's six other kinds of a problem as well.

New-fashioned medical thinking accepts the fact that plain, old everyday overweight is as stubborn, obscure, and complex a problem as doctors and psychiatrists have ever been handed. Yet it can't be dismissed, banal as it is, because it's right at the top of the list of our national health problems.

At a recent gathering of top American obesity experts, Harvard's Dr. Jean Mayer reported that so far, doctors have had little practical success in developing sound reducing diets.

For some patients the next step is the analyst's couch. (Obviously this is not the solution indicated for *all* of America's overweight millions.) Analysts point out firmly that while overweight is often related to neurosis, it can also be the result of external factors. Ignorance about calories is one such external factor. Lack of medical supervision can be another.

But the puzzling fact remains that people who aren't particularly neurotic, who have had good medical care, and who know their calories, still have trouble keeping their weight down.

The answer for many may lie in a third external factor—a factor so big that it's invisible, in exactly the same sense expressed in the saying: "You can't see the wood for the trees."

This factor is what sociologists call "a cultural lag." Fashion and health standards have changed radically since our father's day; but our cooking has not kept pace.

It's scarcely news that we lead far more sedentary lives than our fathers did. We've modernized our menus somewhat. We eat lighter meals.

Yet our recipes have not adjusted to the great changes that have taken place in our living pattern since the beginning of the century. Our cookery is still packed with the highly concentrated ingredients of America's hard early days. And they add little to flavor, though much to fat.

The aim of this book is to adapt the old heavyweight nineteenth-century recipes to our new twentieth century needs, by introducing a *new cooking technology.*

This book concentrates on how to change your weight without changing your habits. It isn't going to try to "reform" you. You can eat, sin, and still get thin . . . after you've read this book. It gives you tangible, tested tools—shopping lists, brand names, menus, recipes—for de-calorizing your family's favorite dishes.

All the recipes are quick, simple, easy. Semiprepared foods are used as much as possible to shorten further the preparation time. With bigger families, less domestic help, and so many women holding jobs outside their homes, it is assumed that much cooking must be done in practically no time.

Since any number of delicious, seemingly complicated recipes are merely variations of certain master recipes, this book teaches mastery of six basic recipes that will help a cook to DE-CALORIZE SEVERAL HUNDRED FAVORITE RECIPES—and fraction their preparation time as well!

America's traditional recipes were not handed down from The Mount; they were compounded, not in laboratories by white-coated technicians, but by ordinary women in gingham aprons with no help but that of their taste buds and imaginations.

We need this kind of creative cook to modernize and de-calorize, using the de-calorized new ingredients food chemists have perfected for us.

De-calorizing the family's favorite dishes takes ingenuity, and it takes doing. But it's an intriguing game, perhaps because it challenges those creative instincts that are the making of a good cook.

This book is intended to act as such a challenge, encouraging good cooks to use their skills and imaginations to carry on from the starting points herein indicated.

Stop
Dieting!
Start
Losing!

I

Like Mother Used to Make—
Minus Calories!

Mrs. America's problem is that her husband and children are often more conservative in their eating habits than she is. She can't *make* them begin to eat a whole strange new way; she'd lose her happy home.

So let's give people the dishes they like, the traditional American favorites, *de-calorized*. They look, taste, and smell "like mother used to make." The only difference is that they contain less calories.

There's a low-calorie version of almost every high-calorie favorite: hot cakes and maple syrup, spaghetti with any old sauce, hot muffins, Yankee pot roast, goulash, roast beef, hamburgers, lamb stew, chop suey, chow-mein, apple pie, chocolate layer cake, sandwiches, ice cream with any kind of slurpy topping.

Thanks to sugarless sweeteners, and to new ways for short-cutting on fats and starches, a willing cook can recreate the family's favorite dishes minus a lethal freight of flavorless calories.

Over a period of time, consistent low-calorie cooking will take off pounds by the rational method of *consistently* lowering the calorie content of your food.

Calorie savings on every dish, every meal, every day, mount up just as reliably as money you put in the bank. Four thousand calories in a pound of fat. By subtracting four thousand calories from your intake

1

every four or five days, you lose considerably more
than a pound of fat (assuming of course that your
metabolism is within normal range). That's because
along with the fat goes water loss.

It's simple to add calories to the servings of de-
calorized dishes for those members of the family who
don't have to think about their weight. They get whole
milk with the meal, extra butter on their vegetables,
gravy on their meat (left with its fat edging). Their
salad dressing comes out of a different jar, and is made
with oil. They get larger servings of dessert—more
nuts, more cream. Their between-meal snacks are calorie-loaded and coupled with milk shakes or eggnogs.

The recipes in this book leave *in* all the calories
that make *goodness* and *vitality,* only leave *out* the
calories that make fat.

Men madden women by losing faster on the same
number of calories. That's because their metabolisms
burn fat faster. Yet most men have a harder time
getting off weight than women. Their lives leave them
much less freedom to edit their food. They lunch out;
they're at the mercy of their wives' cooking at night.
In some circles their manhood is held to depend on a
certain amount of two-fisted drinking. And those alcohol calories are very sneaky to cope with, socially,
psychologically, and physiologically.

Overweight children and adolescents have the
hardest time of all losing those dangerous and unsightly
pounds that set them so painfully apart. To a far
greater degree than adults, they are helpless victims of
emotional tensions (both their own and their parents')
and uninformed eating practices.

What this book is not. It is not a "doctor book."
If you're thirty of forty pounds overweight you ought
to go to a doctor. *It is not primarily a textbook on
nutrition, though the emphasis throughout the book is
on eating for vitality.* Mechanically, overweight is a
nutritional problem. "Whatever Miss T eats, turns into
Miss T," observed the poet Walter de la Mare.

Eating right can lengthen our lives by years. But
it can work far more immediate wonders. If informed

feeding can almost double the healing speed of wounds, if it can increase sexual drive, restore lost potency and fertility, also emotional stability, isn't it worth while to learn *what* it is in what you eat that brings about such results?

What this book is. "Every reducing cure, regardless of whether it is self-elected or recommended by a physician for aesthetic or medical reasons, puts the patient's 'will-power' to a severe test. Invariably the candidate for reducing discovers that he must abstain from his favorite foods. He is constantly tempted by the 'forbidden' food, and therefore fights a never-ending battle," asserts Dr. Edmund S. Bergler in his book, *The Basic Neurosis.*

This book is a *new* kind of reducing cure.

By de-calorizing "the patient's" favorite foods, your calorie intake is reduced and you gradually drop weight. But you aren't on a restricted "diet," so you can't fall *off* it. Your whole effort is to *by-pass* the issue of "forbidden" foods. You want to avoid that battle with your will power which you're so likely to lose. "The only way to win an argument is never to start it," wrote Disraeli.

The obvious effectiveness of this strategy is that it copes with the reducer's biggest hazard—his own psychology.

2

How to Modernize
Your Recipes

FOUR BASIC DE-CALORIZING PROCEDURES

There are two basic procedures by which you cut
calories. First, you leave out certain high-calorie ingredients. Second, you substitute low-calorie ingredients for fattening ones. *But only where you can do so
without noticeably changing either the flavor or the
texture of the finished product.*

This means that it's just as important to know
what to leave in as what to take out. Here are a few
suggestions.

Don't subtract the luxury touches

We eat with our taste buds, placed stingily by
Nature only on the tip, sides, and back of our tongues.
We eat with our eyes. We eat with our palpi, which
gives us our awareness of the textures of food; but
most of all we eat with our noses. In fact, it turns out
that flavor is *mostly* smell. We are told that we can
distinguish some ten thousand odors, but only four
tastes: sour, salt, sweet, and bitter.

But we also eat with our egos. The prestige that
certain foods have gives them special zest: vintage
wines; caviar; truffles; the thick, thick steaks; the thin,
thin tea sandwiches. Food that comes to the table

looking festive and luxurious flatters us—fills emotional needs that are likely to be especially important to people who dearly love to eat.

If your family likes desserts, keep them coming, complete with the gala touches they love. Strew a few chopped nuts on top, slosh on a topping of "whipped cream." Keep the cookie jar full too. And have candy around the house—many kinds are surprisingly low-calorie.

Don't forget the cherry in the grapefruit. Don't forget to float a Parmesan-topped toast round in your onion soup; a dollop of sour cream on the borsch. Make sure there's hollandaise on the broccoli; melted cheese on the broiled tomatoes; plenty of low-calorie mayonnaise for the cold salmon; a few black walnuts in the boiled onions.

Give them treats: a first course of shrimps with cocktail sauce; oysters or clams on the half shell. They're filling, luxurious, and excellent calorie buys.

You can use wine, rum, brandy in your cooking. The heat evaporates the alcohol which is where the calories largely lurk, and only the good flavor is left. Are cherries *flambé* a treat? Have them often. Put a little white wine in your fish sauce, see that a little red wine is cooked with the beef, add a bit of sherry to the creamed chicken. Be sparing of liqueurs served cold on fruit, but use them. A little gives a lot of flavor.

Don't subtract what makes aroma

Lucky for us that it's fragrance, not calories, that is the number one element in most of the dear familiar flavors. Because onions and herbs and vanilla and most of their aromatic friends don't have calories.

Keeping the noses of your family happy is vitally important. Therefore even if an aromatic ingredient has plenty of calories, I would suggest that you put it in. For instance, the grated Parmesan cheese on your spaghetti with meat sauce contains 100 calories an ounce. But it's an essential part of the zest, the strong goodness of the dish, and the object of this game is to keep the deliciousness of the traditional recipes and leave out only the ingredients that add calories *without* adding flavor.

Don't subtract what makes texture interest

Because teeth, tongue, and palpi have so much to do with our enjoyment of food, be conscious of what's creamy, what's crisp, what's chewy, what's firm, what's foamy, and the gradations in between. Mix and contrast them as you do the bland with the sharp, the sweet with the sour. These are the basics of oriental cookery and the best of occidental cookery the world over.

Texture contrast is not only essential to good cooking, it's also a big help in de-calorizing recipes without sacrificing eating fun. Take whipped cream, for instance: 50 calories in a tablespoonful of it. But how much of the pleasure of whipped cream is in its taste and how much is in its foam-velvet texture? Your family will never know the difference if your "whipped cream" is the wonderful new evaporated skimmed milk which whips beautifully when chilled and because it quadruples in volume, contains only 3 calories a tablespoonful, instead of 50. And this low-calorie "whipped cream" is kinder to your food budget than pure cream.

When you can't think of a substitute for texture interest, use the real thing—that's how vital *texture* is to eating pleasure. But use it sparingly and use it where it shows—where the eye can anticipate the pleasure of the palate.

For instance, you shouldn't leave the crisp toasted slivered almonds off your Filet of Sole Amandine. They're the soul of the dish; they look good, they taste luxurious, they're the contrast that raises this fish dish from the humdrum to the heights. And almonds are one of the best calorie buys among nuts —only about 6 calories each.

So think to add the texture contrast of a crunchy something to a creamy dish: croutons, crumbled bacon, chopped celery or raw green pepper, toast crumbs, sliced water chestnuts, chitlings, poppy or sesame seeds; to desserts: finely chopped bitter chocolate, a sprinkle of crushed peanut brittle, crushed hard mints, toasted coconuts, or chopped nuts. They add an exciting dimension to eating pleasure, and open up a whole new bag of fool-the-palate tricks.

Do subtract this

Solid fats. *Nothing* makes you fat as fast as fat. An ounce of sugar or starch is 125 calories; an ounce of whisky or vodka 86 calories. But trim an ounce of *fat* off a steak, and you're trimming off *250 calories*.

Nothing makes you *old* as fast as fat, either. You've heard that hardening of the arteries—arteriosclerosis—is just another name for old age? The lesions of arteriosclerosis are composed principally of cholesterol. (Cholesterol is found in eggs, meat, and dairy products.) The amount of cholesterol itself, taken in the diet, is not now believed to contribute to a high blood level of the subtance. But there is evidence that the amount of solid fat in the diet may be related to the amount of cholesterol in the blood (carbohydrates figure in this too).

Now you need some fat—but not solid fat. What you need is 1 to 2 tablespoons of un-hydrogenated oil a day. Why? Because this is the ONLY big source of lecithin and linoleic acid, two fatty acids essential to life itself. Butter won't give you any to speak of, unfortunately. But the fanciest kind comes built right into corn oil (yes, Mazola) and fish. Other good sources: nuts, avocados, safflower and soybean oil. Look at the label on your salad oil bottle or peanut butter jar. If it says "hydrogenated," that means it won't turn rancid, and you needn't keep it in the refrigerator. BUT also it's got nothing in it but calories! Whereas your 1 to 2 tablespoons of UNhydrogenated oil may actually *help* you lose weight, because

1. It reduces the water held by your tissues
2. It satisfies hunger, reduces cravings for sweets, alcohol

3. It causes your body to change sugar to fat
more slowly

Also, linoleic acid fats helps to protect you against a
high serum cholesterol level and heart ailments.

Trim *all* fat off *all* meat before cooking. "But
you're cutting all the good part off!" the older genera-
tion will wail. It just isn't true. Fat is distributed
throughout the meat fibers. A good steak is marbled
with fat. You can safely trim off every bit of outside
fat, so that it's as clean as a *filet mignon*. If you don't,
remember that enough fat can be sopped up by the
meat to double or triple the original fattening value.
(Look at a *cold* piece of steak, sometime: it's coated
with fat.)

A veal cutlet and a chicken breast aren't streaked
with fat. But their goodness doesn't depend on their
fat but on how they are prepared.

This de-fatting is a completely painless way to
stop dieting and start losing, once you open your mind
to it and adjust your cooking methods. You'll actually
be feeding your family better, because you'll be giving
them only that part of the meat that builds vitality
—the protein calories. What you're depriving them
of—the fat calories—only builds bad figures, diabetes,
arteriosclerosis, heart trouble, and half a dozen other
miseries.

Note: While the amount of fat regular "hamburger" contains is limited by law in most states, you
can depend on it that you can't afford already-ground
hamburger's high fat content if you're watching your
weight. So ask the butcher to trim off all the fat from
your top-of-the-round steak, before he grinds it for
you. And since this is against a butcher's conservative
grain, ask him to show it to you before he puts it in the
machine. Chances are he's left on two or three ounces
of fat (at 250 calories an ounce, remember).

Do change these

Substitute low-calorie ingredients for fattening
ones.

Instead of flour you use cottage cheese or stiffly

beaten egg whites in muffins, cakes, cookies, pastry (see Basic Recipes).

This isn't as revolutionary as it sounds. Women have been making "cheese pastry" for years. And one of the aristocrats among cakes—angel food—is built on the egg-whites-for-flour principle. Using egg whites has several advantages. Because they're tender, they don't require fat to keep the finished product from being tough or hard. Because they add far more bulk than flour, you get, for instance, 16 muffins from a recipe that, made only with flour, produces 12 muffins. (Twenty-six calories a muffin, instead of 126 —see recipe on page 18.)

Instead of sugar use Sucaryl (sodium cyclamate). You'll find that this book is written as if the wonderful cyclamates (sugar's *only* match for taste) were available . . . as they have been most of the twenty-two years since this book was first published. I've left cyclamates in because they may well be back on the market soon. (Until they are, use saccharine where Sucaryl is called for. Try to avoid *heating* it.) About Sucaryl . . .

All the evidence from the testing and re-testing that has gone on since the almost overnight ban on cyclamates in 1969 points to their utter harmlessness.

This had been clinically well established by the fact that millions of people have consumed cyclamates —without restriction—over two decades. And there hasn't been a single instance of harmful reaction.

Let us fervently hope that the incalculably harmful error in judgment that the ban on cyclamates represents may soon be corrected. It has imposed untold hardship on the millions of us who have diabetes or are predisposed to overweight and its whole life-shortening train of diseases.

This remarkable no-calorie sweetener can do as much for weight-watchers as the wheel did for travel. It's pure gold, and its possibilities are infinite.

Don't be frightened by the stern phrase on the label, "for use only in sugar-restricted diets." (Your doctor will tell you this means *you!*) It's there because of one of those legal donnybrooks. Unlike saccharin, it leaves no bitter after-taste, used moderately either in cooking, or dissolved in your cup of coffee. And it can have no ill effects, no matter how lavishly you use it.

The ultraconservative Abbott Laboratories who make it, have fed people staggering doses, and the worst it can do, taken in massive amounts, is to act as a mild laxative.

You can buy powdered Sucaryl, too. It comes in a shaker-topped bottle. It is more expensive, but fine for cereal and fruit. I transfer mine to a pretty sugar-shaker I can keep on the table. It's also available in liquid form but this is an expensive way to buy it. It's very easy to make the liquid form yourself because it dissolves fizzily in hot water.

Each Sucaryl tablet equals a teaspoon of sugar in sweetening power. Make up a bottleful of liquid and have it handy for quick use. To a cupful of hot water, dissolve forty-eight tablets, then each teaspoon-ful of the liquid will equal a teaspoon of sugar; each tablespoon, a tablespoon; and the cupful of liquid, a cupful of sugar.

For cooking, you'll usually want far more concentrated solutions, but you can vary the concentration as much as you choose.

In cooking it's a calorie-saver beyond your wildest dreams. Take cranberry sauce, for instance. The recipe in your cookbook calls for 1½ cups of sugar to a pound of cranberries. For the cranberries, 218 calories; for the sugar, 1,155 calories! These sugar calories are hidden calories, because your sauce will be just as freshly sweet, just as tangily good, if you use Sucaryl for almost all the sweetening.

You can't always use Sucaryl entirely in place of sugar; but you *can* cut your week's total calorie intake enormously by substituting Sucaryl as often as you can—and that's far oftener than you'd dream, till you try.

If your family has a mouthful of sweet teeth, the existence of Sucaryl in the world will enable you to melt pounds off them without a pang. And before

Sucaryl, this addiction to sweets was the hurdle few "fatties" could get over—especially children.

Instead of fat, less fat, or bouillon. All fats are equally fattening *ounce for ounce*: margarine (diet margarines are fluffed with water), butter, vegetable oil. There is no low-calorie fat. They're all 250 calories per ounce. The only no-calorie fat is mineral oil, and that interferes with absorption of vitamin A and possibly vitamins E, D, and K.

However, in editing traditional recipes you'll find that very often you can use much less fat than is called for. Often you don't need any fat at all. For example, consider the two or three tablespoonfuls of fat automatically called for in browning meat, sautéing chopped onions, etc. You'll see that the onions will wilt just as delectably—and more flavorfully—in a little bouillon. The merest film of oil is all that's required to seal in meat juices.* Spray the pan with vegetable oil. If you're using a properly heavy pan so that the heat is distributed gradually and evenly, you'll get just as good results. Or use a Teflon-type pan. Or brown meat under the broiler. Quick, easy—no fat required.

Instead of whipped cream, you can almost always use the non-dairy whipped toppings: Bird's Eye Cool Whip (14 calories per tablespoon); Dream Whip. Look for others, they're firm, fluffy, almost too sweet in some instances (I use Kirsch to cut that sweetness and add a twist of flavor).

You may whip dry skimmed milk. Fine for last-minute whipped topping. And cottage cheese whips to a beautiful thick "cream" in your electric mixer; is the basis for hollandaise, frostings and dressings. You'll see as you read on.

And add these:

Use the new de-calorized processed foods and drink, available for the calorie-conscious. Almost every

---

*Rub the merest film of oil on the back of your hand. Drop water on the oiled surface. See for yourself how effectively a film of oil *seals* moisture out. *Or inl*

month a new de-calorized item hits the market, or an improved version of an old product. So keep trying and spying and buying for what's new in health stores, department stores, and in the dietetic sections of your supermarket.

3

Six Twentieth-Century
Master Recipes

Just as there are reputed to be only about six basic jokes in the world, a good part of any cuisine boils down largely to about six basic recipes. Any number of delectable, seemingly complicated dishes are merely variations of these master recipes.

Once you have perfected the low-calorie versions of these six recipes, you can improvise on them endlessly.

TWENTIETH-CENTURY MASTER RECIPE NO. 1

De-fatted "Cream" Sauce—
for casseroles, sauces, etc.

A cream sauce or white sauce is the foundation of literally hundreds of our best-loved dishes. Because it's so handy in making main dishes out of leftovers, it's one of your budget's best friends, too.

But it's horribly fattening—27 calories in one level tablespoon; 430 calories in a cupful. If you use part *cream,* about 600 calories in a cup.

The lack of a low-calorie cream sauce has limited the good eating of dieters perhaps more than any other one missing link. It's fattening and it's bothersome to make. Many women consider it one of the persnicketi-

13

est jobs a cook has. They won't be bothered. They use the cream soups that come in cans.

But if you're watching your weight—look out! That can of condensed cream of mushroom soup holds 330 calories—and you'll have to add more milk calories to dilute it.

Wouldn't it be wonderful to find a low-calorie "cream" sauce that you could whisk together in three minutes—foolproof, sinfully rich-tasting, and only, say, 5 calories per tablespoon? Well, here it is.

3-MINUTE DE-FATTED "CREAM" SAUCE
Only 51 calories per cupful
versus 430 calories made traditionally

		calories
2 tablespoons cake flour		46
4 tablespoons instant dry milk powder		112
1 teaspoon flavor salt (preferably Lawry's Seasoned Salt)		
¼ teaspoon salt		
½ teaspoon monosodium glutamate		
⅛ teaspoon pepper		
2 cups water		
	total	158 for 2 cups

Put the 2 cups of water in your electric blender. Dump the rest of the ingredients on top. put the cover on the blender and turn it on top speed. Run it a minute—until the mix is a foamy cream. Empty liquid into heavy aluminum pan. Over high heat, stir constantly with a spatula, using the flat wide end of the spatula to keep mixture from sticking to bottom of pan. The sauce will be bubbling, thick and perfectly smooth in 2 minutes.

This low-calorie cream sauce has a cozy taste, creamy, fragrant, and savory.

If you like, melt in a tablespoon of grated sharp Cheddar cheese. The "cost" is only 14 calories more per cup. This isn't enough to make it taste like a cheese sauce, but only adds a pleasantly buttery flavor.

Or add a tablespoon of sherry after you take the

sauce off the stove. Very few more calories, and a pleasant taste-twist. If you're a fusser, a few drops of yellow vegetable coloring is a good *trompe-l'oeil* idea when you use the sauce as a topping where it's right in the spotlight.

If you like a thicker "medium cream sauce" than this, start with an extra tablespoon of flour in the dry mix. Add 12 calories to the count per cup.

Uses for medium cream sauce

For anything creamed: use as is; or plus the herbs or flavorings suggested in your favorite cookbooks for creamed *vegetables;* such as onions, carrots, asparagus, peas, potatoes, chopped spinach; for creamed *fish,* such as codfish, tunafish, finnan haddie; for creamed *meats,* such as creamed chipped beef, chicken or turkey.

For anything scalloped: such as potatoes, corn, eggplant, etc.; *fish,* such as oysters or clams; *eggs,* hard-boiled, shelled, and sliced. Directions: In a lightly oiled casserole, arrange the food prepared for serving, and the cream sauce, in layers. Top with a sprinkling of cheese or toast crumbs. Bake in a moderate oven (375°) about 25 minutes, or until browned.

For anything deviled: such as crab meat, lobster, clams, oysters. To cream sauce, add ½ cup sharp Cheddar cheese, grated; 1 teaspoon Worchestershire sauce; dash of cayenne. Follow directions in your pet cookbook for assembling the dish.

For anything au gratin: such as sliced potatoes, cauliflower, cabbage, sliced hard-cooked eggs, mushrooms, salmon, fish fillets. In a shallow, oiled baking dish, place food ready for serving. Add 1 teaspoon of minced parsley to cream sauce and 3 tablespoons sharp Cheddar cheese, grated. Pour over food; sprinkle with grated cheese. Bake in 375° oven until browned.

For anything à la king: such as chicken, turkey, eggs, ham. Add to the cream sauce 1 medium green pepper, minced; 1 pimento, diced; ½ cup sliced mushrooms; 1 tablespoon sherry.

For anything curried: such as chicken, lamb, lobster, shrimp, beef, hard-boiled eggs. Add to the cream sauce 2 teaspoons curry; 1½ teaspoons sugar; ¼ cup minced onion; 1 tart green apple, peeled and chopped; 1 teaspoon chopped candied ginger. Just before serving, stir in 2 tablespoons fresh lime or lemon juice.

Other variations:

Sauce Newburg: for lobster, crab, mixed sea food. Add 2 well-beaten egg yolks to cream sauce, a few grains of nutmeg, a few grains of cayenne. Just before serving, stir in ⅓ cup of sherry.

Cheese sauce: Stir 6 tablespoons sharp Cheddar, grated, and ½ teaspoon Worcestershire sauce into finished sauce. Continue cooking, stirring constantly over low heat until cheese is melted. Good with macaroni, potatoes, rice, eggs, tomatoes.

Thick "cream sauce" for soufflés

Prepare as directed for de-fatted cream sauce (see page 14) using 6 tablespoons of flour instead of 2. Increase instant dry milk to 6 tablespoons, also.

Cheese Soufflé

Traditional recipe (makes 4 to 6 servings)

	calories
1 cup thick cream sauce	590
1½ cups, grated, processed Cheddar cheese	839
few grains cayenne	
4 eggs separated	304
total	1,733

Low-calorie version (makes 4 to 6 servings)

1 cup de-fatted thick cream sauce	165
¼ pound natural sharp Cheddar cheese, grated	451
2 tablespoons Parmesan Cheese, grated	40
½ teaspoon Worcestershire sauce	
2 egg yolks	122
4 egg whites	60
¼ teaspoon salt	
¼ teaspoon cream tartar	
total	838

To the hot cream sauce, add cheeses, Worcestershire sauce, and stir over low heat until cheese is melted; remove from heat. Fold a little of the sauce into the well-beaten yolks. Fold into remaining sauce.

Sprinkle salt on egg whites, which should be at room temperature. Beat until foamy. Sprinkle cream of tartar on egg whites and beat until stiff but not dry. Fold into cheese mixture.

Pour into a casserole brushed very lightly with oil. Casserole should not be more than half full.

Bake in a preheated slow oven (300°) about half an hour. Serve immediately.

Here you save calories by using cheeses which have more concentrated flavor and aroma for less calories, and skipping a couple of egg yolks which don't turn out to be necessary for texture's sake; nor for color. Also there's the big initial saving your de-fatted cream sauce gives you.

Dione Lucas uses 2 wedges of Camembert cheese, instead of Cheddar, in her *The Cordon Bleu Cookbook's* cheese soufflé. Camembert gives a very good flavor and is even lower calorie than natural Cheddar.

Adele Davis's excellent cookbook tartly entitled *Cook It Right,* explains, scientifically yet simply, exactly what makes a soufflé stand or fall . . . and why you'll do well to serve soufflés often. She also suggests many soufflé variations which you can use, starting from this low-calorie basic recipe. *Cook It Right* is a good book to have—full of fine nutritional lowdown.

TWENTIETH-CENTURY MASTER RECIPE NO. 2

Muffins

Traditional Recipe (makes 12 muffins)	*calories*
2 cups flour	728
3 teaspoons baking powder	
¾ teaspoon salt	
3 tablespoons sugar	146
1 egg	76
1 cup milk	170
4 tablespoons shortening	400
total	1,520
each muffin	126

De-fatted recipe (makes 16 muffins)	
1 cup flour	364
3 teaspoons baking powder	
½ teaspoons salt	
1 teaspoon cinnamon	
5 tablespoons water	
1 teaspoon grated orange peel	
5 egg whites	75
1 teaspoon cream of tartar	144
3 tablespoons sugar	
¼ teaspoon almond flavoring	
total	583
each muffin	36

Sift flour; measure; add baking powder, cinnamon, salt; sift again. (Here's where you add nuts, dates, or blueberries, etc. And *do!*)

To unbeaten egg whites, add the water. Don't worry; they'll beat until just stiff. Beat in sugar. Fold dry mix lightly into egg whites. Just as stiff, *twice* as big! Sprinkle on a little salt, cream of tartar. Beat, add orange peel, flavoring. Quickly fill oiled muffin tins *full*. Bake in preheated oven (375°). Serve hot (or re-heat).

The calorie saving on this de-fatted muffin recipe is sensational, and you'll get no complaints on the muffins. The crusts are a rich golden brown; the grain uniform, with moist tender crumbs. Just the faintest whiff of cinnamon and orange can be detected by Hawkshaw taste buds.

You'll notice that the method is merely a transposition of the angel-cake principle—using low-calorie egg whites instead of high-calorie, starchy flour for bulk. This recipe is endearingly easy on the family budget, because these egg whites are *free,* if you remember that an egg yolk can behave like a whole egg in many dishes, including scrambled eggs.

Put whipped butter on the table when you serve these muffins. Because there's more air in whipped butter, it's slightly less caloric. Also, it spreads thinner, if you cooperate! Instead of jam, try cinnamon and sugar (only 18 calories per teaspoon—saves calories).

However, a far shrewder way to save calories, is to serve those muffins with Sucaryl-sweetened jellies and jams—instead of butter. They have a negligible calorie count—so load 'em on!

Variations (and why not, at these low-calorie prices?):

Blueberry muffins: To sifted dry ingredients add 1 cup fresh blueberries or huckleberries (only 6 calories per muffin).

Raisin muffins: To sifted dry ingredients add ½ cup of raisins (215 calories—still only 49 calories for a whole raisin muffin).

Date muffins: Same procedure as for raisin muffins (same calorie count, about).

Nut muffins: To sifted dry ingredients, add ½ cup of coarsely chopped black or English walnuts (190 calories—but still under 50 calories for a very festive muffin indeed).

Corn muffins: Follow de-fatted master muffin recipe, but substitute for half the flour, ½ cup of yellow corn meal, and increase the baking powder to 3½ teaspoons (same calorie count, approximately).

If you're a muffin-maker, you can go on almost

indefinitely to compound your own; corn-bacon-onion muffins, date-nut-bran muffins, cheese-bacon muffins, banana-nut muffins.

TWENTIETH-CENTURY MASTER RECIPE NO. 3

Jiffy Waffles

40 calories in each crisp, airy waffle
versus 215 calories for a traditional waffle

De-calorized recipe
(makes 10 waffles, or 15 pancakes)

	calories
¾ cup cake flour	300
2 teaspoons baking powder	
¼ teaspoon salt	
¾ cup skimmed milk	66
2 egg whites	30
	total 396

Sprinkle dash of salt on egg whites and beat until stiff, but not dry. Put the milk in blender; just dump the flour and salt on top. Beat until smooth (saves all that tiresome sifting!). Add baking powder. Beat a few seconds. Pour batter quickly into a bowl and fold egg whites lightly into it. Wasn't that easy? And these waffles are *so* good . . . best recipe in the book!

Cook until crisp, *nut-brown,* in preheated waffle iron, without stirring the batter. These take extra-long cooking: leave them in; even after the iron stops steaming. Serve with low calorie maple syrup (from your supermarket) or cinnamon sugar.

Puff Pancakes, 26 calories apiece instead of 60, as in traditional pancake recipe.

Spoon waffle batter (above) onto medium hot griddle. When puffed up and bubbles begin to break, brown on other side. Makes about 15 pancakes, twice as high, twice as light, rich in flavor, and with a chiffon cake texture. Never soggy inside, but fluffy and delightful all the way through. The flavor of the maple "syrup" melts right down in. Or find almost no-calorie sugarless maple syrup in the dietetic section of your supermarket.

TWENTIETH-CENTURY MASTER RECIPE NO. 4

Hollandaise for Moderns

Vital Nutritional *Statistics:*	*Grams of Fat*	*Protein*	*calories*
Hollandaise for Moderns:	2	49.6	351
Same amount, traditional recipe:	248	18.1	1,250

	calories
1 scant cup cottage cheese	215
3 tablespoons lemon juice	16
2 egg yolks	120
½ teaspoon Lawry's Seasoned Salt	
½ teaspoon salt	
dash of pepper	
dash of cayenne	
total	351

Into an electric blender put the cottage cheese, seasonings and lemon juice. Whip until the mixture is a smooth cream. Remove from blender. Stir in egg yolks. Cook, stirring constantly with flat end of spatula, over low heat in a heavy aluminum pan or in double boiler, until just thick. Don't boil. Makes 1¼ cups.

This is a more stable hollandaise than the traditional kind; there's less danger of curdling and separation. It's golden, fluffy, delicately tart. It's just as good cold, as hot. See page 104. You may like a slightly less lemony sauce, but try it this way the first time. Add ¼ teaspoon yellow vegetable coloring, if you like.

If there wasn't any other reason for investing in an electric mixer or blender, this spectacular hollandaise is enough—*if* you like hollandaise. And note how pleasantly inexpensive this twentieth-century version is.

Now you can afford to have this luxurious exciting sauce as often as the fancy takes you.

VARIATIONS:

Dill Hollandaise: Add 1 to 1½ teaspoons fresh dill. Serve with boiled lamb or veal.

Mint Hollandaise: Add 1 teaspoon finely chopped fresh mint. Serve with roast lamb.

Chive Hollandaise: Add 1 tablespoon chopped chives. Serve with meat or vegetables.

Béarnaise Sauce: Decrease lemon juice to 2 tablespoons and add 1 tablespoon tarragon vinegar. Add ½ teaspoon onion powder with seasonings. When sauce is thick add ½ teaspoon chopped fresh tarragon and ¼ teaspoon chopped parsley or chervil.

TWENTIETH-CENTURY MASTER RECIPE NO. 5

Quick, Foolproof Pastry

Only 333 Calories per 1-Crust Pie
Versus 999 Calories for the Traditional 1-Crust Version!

Use the Homogenized Pie Crust Mix. (It comes in two sticks, in some markets. Ask your market manager to stock it, if he doesn't carry it.)

	calories
⅓ of 1 stick (½ ounce)	233
½ cup farmer cheese or pot cheese	100
total	333

(You may substitute cottage cheese but squeeze it dry.) In 8-inch pie pan blend cheese and mix with fork. For fun and flavor add 1 teaspoon sesame seeds. Or grated lemon rind, or Cheddar. When all is well-blended and smooth, pick dough up and work into a ball.

Handling won't toughen this pastry. Flatten into a round cake. Then roll out, on a well-floured surface, into a round, 1 inch larger than the inverted pie pan. Ease the round into the pan—the same one you mixed the dough in. Trim and moisten edge, flute to edge of pan. No matter how you re-roll dough, the pastry won't toughen.

This pastry takes longer baking than usual. It's well to pre-bake bottom crust at 425° for 10 minutes before adding pie filling.

This makes a tender, crisp, delectable pie crust, firm enough to hold any filling, and lift out. It has a clean nutty flavor; contains almost *3 times* the protein and calcium, and is ⅓ *as fattening* as the old heavyweight pastry.

If you roll the dough thin enough, you'll have enough left over to make a few strips to lattice over the top. You can "patch" bits and pieces together without any fear that the pastry will suffer. If you haven't enough left for strips, make little flat "polka dots" of the dough and spot them around on the filling; or cut out fancy little designs (stars and crescents) with a pastry cutter or knife.

Besides using this pastry for pies, tarts, patty shells, turnovers, you can use it to make festive small pastries, such as cocktail cheese sticks, shoofly pastry snacks, Swedish nut wafers, especially come Christmastime when lots of crisp little cookies and pastries in fancy cut-out shapes are called for. One recipe containing 200 calories can make a powerful lot of pastry snacks; if you cut them pretty, cut them small. I haven't tried a puff-paste, but I don't see why it shouldn't work—why don't you try it?

Here are a few pie recipes. Using them as patterns, there's almost no pie that can defy you.

All calorie counts, both de-calorized and traditional, are for ⅐ of an 8-inch pie—approximately a 4-inch sector.

Pumpkin Pie: 123 calories per serving
versus 263 calories in traditional recipe

  2 eggs
  ½ cup sugar
  1 teaspoon cinnamon
  ½ teaspoon ginger
  ¼ teaspoon cloves
  ¼ teaspoon nutmeg
  ½ teaspoon maple flavor
16 Sucaryl tablets
1½ cups skimmed milk
1½ cups pumpkin, canned
     or home-cooked, drained

Mix spices into eggs and beat mixture. Add
sugar and maple flavor. Dissolve Sucaryl in hot
milk. Stir into pumpkin. Warm. Combine with
egg mix. Pour gently into partly pre-baked crust.
Bake in hot oven 425° for 30 to 40 minutes.

Blueberry Pie: 113 calories per serving
versus 291 calories in traditional recipe

2 cups fresh blueberries
¼ cup lemon juice
2 tablespoons sugarless lemon "pop"
8 Sucaryl tablets
¼ cup sugar
2 tablespoons cornstarch
1 teaspoon cinnamon
2 tablespoons water

Bring lemon juice and water to a boil, dissolve Sucaryl tablets in it. Add to blueberries.
Mix sugar, cornstarch, cinnamon, lemon "pop,"
then add blueberry mixture. Pour into partly
pre-baked pie crust. Bake.

Blueberry pie à la mode: Top with low-
calorie ice cream (page 110), 153 calories per
serving.

Apple Pie: 106 or 147 calories
versus 331 calories in traditional recipe

4 cups apples, peeled and sliced
2 tablespoons lemon juice
1 cup No-Cal Creme soda
2 envelopes Dietetic butterscotch pudding mix
1 tablespoon flour
1 teaspoon cinnamon
⅛ teaspoon salt
1 or 2 recipes pastry, de-calorized

Add lemon juice to apples. Dump dry pudding mix from both envelopes into your electric blender with the "pop" and whip at high speed a minute or two.

Mix together flour, cinnamon, and salt, and combine with apples. Arrange apples in pre-baked crust and pour pudding mixture over. Fit upper crust or arrange strips or dots of leftover dough. Bake. (Try maple flavoring instead of cinnamon—good!)

TWENTIETH-CENTURY MASTER RECIPE NO. 6

Basic Cake and Cookie Mixes

ANGEL FOOD CAKE MIX

Angel food cake mix is a boon to weight-watchers. It contains no fat, a minimum of flour, makes *umpteen* cakes, 100 to 140 calories per slice vs. 300 to 500 in traditional cakes. A 2-inch sector of angel food cake contains only a little over 100 calories, as compared to plain foundation cake, which contains almost double the number of calories per serving. And angel food contains twice as much protein as any other kind of cake.

Make cupcakes of it—bake it in loaves or sheets, using the low-calorie frostings and fillings in this chapter.

ANGEL FOOD CAKE MIX VARIATIONS

Cakes and cookies made from this base stay moist and fresh for days, in Saran wrap, aluminum foil or an airtight container. This isn't an expensive cake. It's quick to make; the job is done in two steps. And there's almost no limit to the variety of cakes and cookies you can make out of that one box of low-calorie magic. You add at the most a couple of hundred calories to the whole cake in any of the variations, which amounts to only about 14 calories a serving.

You can bake angel food in layers, too. Divide the batter three ways, use layer-cake tins. Try the sponge cake variation in layers too (see below). Then fill and frost with de-calorized chocolate recipe (see page 31) and you have that No. 1 darling of desserts, a piece of *chocolate layer cake for 140 calories,* instead of the 350 or 400 calories the traditional recipe costs you.

My idea of cake is that there should be just about as much frosting as cake. So I make four thin layers. And I make a lemon or chocolate filling (see page 31) for between layers. This allows me to pile all the icing outside, making a most imposing and delectable production. The moist, tangy filling adds so few calories per piece that you can forget to count them. For texture, garnish! With crushed peanut brittle, mints, or chopped nuts: grated orange rind, coconut or chocolate.

Sunshine Sponge Cake: Measure into a large mixing bowl 1 cup (minus 2 tablespoons) water and 1 teaspoon vanilla. Add egg-white mix from package. Mix slowly with rotary egg beater, flat wire whip, or at low speed of electric mixer until all egg-white powder is moistened.

Then beat vigorously by hand, or at highest speed of electric mixer, until the fluffy whites form stiff peaks when beater is raised. Sprinkle in 3 tablespoons sugar and beat about 10 seconds longer. Set aside.

Sift flour mixture into small bowl. Add 3 unbeaten egg yolks, 1½ teaspoons grated lemon rind, and ¼ cup water. Beat until just blended—about ½ minute.

Fold into the stiffly beaten egg whites with about 40 fold-over strokes, using a spoon or wire whip.

Turn batter into ungreased 9½ or 10-inch tube

pan. Bake in pre-heated moderate oven (375°) 35 minutes, or until cake springs back when pressing lightly.

Cool cake in pan, upside-down on wire rack, until cold—1 to 2 hours. Then loosen from sides and center of pan with knife and gently remove cake.

Chocolate Angel Cake: Prepare angel food cake mix as directed on package, increasing water to 1⅓ cups and sifting 3 tablespoons cocoa with last ¼ of flour mix. Fold carefully until well blended. If desired, fold in ½ cup finely chopped nuts, before pouring into pan.

Chocolate Chip Angel Cake: Prepare angel food cake mix as directed on package. Fold in 2 squares (2 ounces) semi-sweet chocolate, grated, before pouring into pan.

Marble Cake: Sift 1 tablespoon cocoa with 5 tablespoons of flour mix. Mix batter for angel food cake as directed on package, using balance of flour mix. Place ¼ of batter in second bowl; fold in cocoa mixture. Sprinkle white and dark batter alternately into pan.

Upside-down Cake: In cake pan, prepare one of the toppings below. Then make cake as label directs. Carefully turn batter over topping. Bake at 375° F. 40 to 50 minutes or until well done. Cool in pan on wire rack 10 minutes; then invert, fruit side up, on serving plate. Let stand 1 minute, lift off pan. Serve slightly warm, with or without whipped milk, ice cream, or whipped cottage cheese. Two cakes to a package; 100 calories in each big serving!

Nutted Apricot: In 9 x 9 x 2-inch pan, melt 1 tablespoon butter or margarine. Over it, sprinkle ¼ cup granulated or brown sugar. Arrange on top, with cut sides down, 1 can Diet-Sweet apricot halves, drained (or use fresh fruit). Sprinkle with ½ cup coarsely chopped nuts.

Pineapple Chunk: In 9 x 9 x 2-inch pan, melt 1 tablespoon butter or margarine. Over it sprinkle ¼

cup brown sugar. Arrange 1 Dole Dietetic can pineapple, drained, on top. Nice with gingerbread or gin-
ger-cake mix, too.

QUICK TRICKS WITH STORE-BOUGHT SPONGE
OR ANGEL CAKES

Ice Cream Cake: Turn cake upside-down. Enlarge
the hole in the center by cutting out one inch of
cake from the center. Fill with softened de-calorized
ice cream. (See page 112.) Immediately wrap carefully with freezer weight paper such as aluminum foil,
cellophane, pliofilm. Freeze until firm and serve immediately.

If in freezer overnight or longer, allow about ½
hour in refrigerator for cake to thaw. Before serving,
cover sides and top with sweetened whipped skimmed
evaporated milk or Choc-Low. Sprinkle chopped nuts
over top, if desired.

Coconut Balls: Cut left-over angel food cake into
pieces about two-inch square. Gently mold into
rounded shape. Dip into and cover with any filling
on pages 31–2. Roll in moist shredded coconut. Icing
may be tinted, if desired.

COOKIES

Nutty Brownies: under 70 calories each versus
200 calories for traditional recipe.

Prepare angel food cake mix according to directions. Just before spreading batter in thin sheets in
large square pans, add 1 7-ounce jar of Choc-Low
and 1 cup of coarsely cut-up English walnut meats.
Make 30 fudgy, chewy brownies.

Date-Nut Bars: 80 calories each versus 180 calories for traditional recipe. Make angel food cake mix
according to directions. For baking, spread batter in
thin sheets in large square pans. On the surface dot
¾ cup of coarsely ground English walnuts, ¾ cup of
quartered pitted dates. After baking dust lightly with
powdered sugar before cutting bars. Makes 30 bars.

GINGERBREAD MIX

A versatile calorie buy and only 88 calories per square.

A package of Pillsbury's Gingerbread Mix, you will be happy to learn, contains only around 1,390 calories. (Other brands I checked contain 200 or 300 more.)

And a-h-h, the satisfying titillation of hot gingerbread's flavor and aroma! The delightful assault on one's senses of that giant ginger fragrance, the ardent bite of ginger's taste on the tongue! Bake it in a 9 x 9 x 2-inch pan and you can cut it in 16 pieces: 88 calories per square. Serve as a dessert. It deserves the center of the stage.

Six fragrant, hot gingerbread desserts
—quick, big and easy
Only 105 to 130 calories in each fat serving

1. Just squares of hot gingerbread—split and spread with butterscotch filling (page 32) and topped with chopped nuts.
2. Pile sweetened whipped dry skimmed milk flavored with lemon on a hot gingerbread square, then grate fresh orange peel over it.
3. This is one of my favorites: again, just a square of hot ginger bread, but in between and on top, lots of quick-prepared lemon pudding (the de-calorized kind, of course).
4. Ice-cream sandwiches: Cut gingerbread into pieces the size of Zwieback. On top and in between two pieces of gingerbread, put slices of de-calorized ice cream. Serve with butterscotch sauce. (Make up D-Zerta sugar-free butterscotch pudding to directions on package for this.)
5. Pineapple Cream: Whip 1 can chilled evaporated milk. Fold in 2 tablespoons confectioners' sugar, ¾ cup Dole's Dietetic crushed pineapple, well drained, and 1 tablespoon maraschino cherries cut in quarters and well drained. Serve on squares of warm gingerbread.

6. Banana Cream: Whip 1 can chilled evaporated milk with 2 tablespoons lemon juice until stiff. Fold in ¼ cup *sifted* confectioners' sugar. Spoon on warm gingerbread squares and place banana slices on end in whipped milk.

GINGER DROP COOKIES

Only 25 calories in each—these are so easy a child can make them.

Into contents of package stir 1 teaspoon ginger. Dissolve 24 Sucaryl tablets in ½ cup hot water. Mix this into 1½ cups of pot cheese or cottage cheese, drained dry. Combine into a smooth batter. Chill.

Heat oven to 375°. Drop by teaspoons onto lightly oiled cookie sheet. Bake 15 minutes. Makes 75 cookies.

These cookies are crisp outside, chewily tender inside, and of a warm spiciness that's hard to beat. Vary them by adding black walnut flavoring to the batter, and ½ cup of black walnut meats. Adds about 5 calories to each cookie. Or put a quarter of an English walnut on top of each cookie before baking. Or a chunk of date.

ROLLED GINGER COOKIES

25 calories each.

Follow directions in previous recipe, only use ⅓ cup of water instead of ½ cup. Chill 1 to 2 hours. Heat oven to 375°. Roll dough ⅛ inch thick on floured cloth-covered board. Cut with floured cookie cutter; place on lightly oiled cookie sheet. Bake 12 to 15 minutes.

Come Christmas, like the petit fours, this is a fine basic strategy for fancy Christmas cookies, cut in stars and crescents and Santa Clauses and Christmas trees. (Naturally the number of calories will depend on the size of the cookie.)

Sprinkle each Christmas cookie with colored sugars and/or tiny candies. There's a Virginia Dare line

of these in sparkling colors. Chocolate sprinkles make
a good garnish too; or a chip of candied orange peel
or candied ginger; or dust with powdered sugar.

Or drop a tiny whirl of frosting on each, out of a
pastry tube or off a teaspoon, frosting made by moistening confectioner's sugar with lemon juice and stirring
into a paste. Make this a thin paste and you can ice
each cookie all over without adding many calories.

De-Calorized Cake-Fillings, Toppings
*3-minute Lemon Filling, 57 calories per cup,
versus 911 traditionally.*

- 1 tablespoon lemon juice
- 1⅓ cups sugarless lemon soda (Cott, Hoffman, No-Cal)
- 2 envelopes D-Zerta sugar-free vanilla pudding
- 2 envelopes D-Zerta sugar-free lemon gelatin
- 1 tablespoon cornstarch (first mixed with a little water)

In electric blender, blend all. In heavy
aluminum pan, bring to a boil, stirring with flat
end of spatula. Chill until set, before spreading.

*Whipped Cream Filling or Topping, 60 calories
a cup, versus 500 traditionally.*

- ¼ cup No-Cal Creme soda (has a vanilla flavor)
- 1 tablespoon lemon juice
- 2 tablespoons dry skimmed milk
- ½ teaspoon unflavored gelatin

Beat all in small bowl until stiff, with electric
beater. Chill.

Lemon Cream Filling or Topping: Fold
cooled lemon filling into whipping cream filling.
Chill.

*Chocolate filling, 69 calories per recipe
versus 2,320 made traditionally!* Whip together
in electric blender 1⅓ cups No-Cal Creme soda,
2 envelopes D-Zerta chocolate pudding, 1 teaspoon unflavored gelatin, 4 teaspoons Choc-Low,

1 tablespoon cornstarch. Cook (see lemon filling). Chill.

Chocolate Cream Filling: Fold into cream filling.

Butterscotch filling: Follow recipe for chocolate filling, substituting D-Zerta butterscotch pudding for chocolate. Add 1 teaspoon butterscotch flavoring.

Butterscotch cream filling: Fold into whipped cream filling.

"Cool-Whip," already prepared, in your supermarket is only 14 calories per tablespoon. You'll need to add a sharp flavoring to it: peppermint, or Jamaica rum, or bourbon.

4

The New Phantom Foods

WHAT TO LOOK FOR; WHAT TO LOOK OUT FOR; PLUS A LIST OF DE-CALORIZED FOODS— WITH SHOPPING SOURCES

With about three people out of four keeping an eye on the scales today, there's scarcely a supermarket or department store in the country without its special section of "dietetic foods." Advertisements in every newspaper and magazine you pick up shout: "Less fattening than—" or "Absolutely nonfattening—" and so on. You'd like to believe every word of it, but the extravagance and number of claims and counterclaims leave you confused and skeptical. Who, and what, can one believe? How can one tell the valid claims from the phony ones?

The seamy side!

If you have done some browsing around in your supermarket's dietetic food section, you've probably been appalled, too, at how expensive a lot of the low-calorie items are. And even in a big dietetic food section you don't see enough different items to make up a menu for even one meal, to say nothing of three meals a day for days and weeks and months. Also, you've probably had the experience of buying some of those dietetic foods, and then when you got them home and sampled them—ouch! They were about as edible as sawdust!

How to pick the winners

Here are the four operating principles which will enable you to pick the good nutrition and calorie buys, not just in the dietetic food section, but *all over your pet supermarket*. And there are hundreds of these low-calorie food favorites, as you will see by the shopping check list for weight-watchers which you will find at the end of this chapter.

Principle one: Keep your nutritional ABC's firmly in mind and favor foods that are high in protein, low in "empty" calories. This means starch, fats, and sugar. (Anything that ends in "ose" is just another form of sugar—dextrose, maltose, sucrose, glucose. There are about a hundred of these substances under various names.)

Principle two: Carry your calorie counter and check calorie values.

Principle three: Read all that tiny print on the package label. Somewhere you will find all the ingredients listed. And you'll find the net weight of the package contents printed on the package somewhere. From these two items, you can pretty well calculate the calorie and nutritional values. Exact calorie content will usually be printed on products carried in the dietetic food section.

Principle four: Don't let a few disappointments put you off your search for favorite foods that are also low in calories. Old stand-bys, now miraculously decalorized, are to be found in that dietetic food section. And every week you'll find new items and improved versions of old ones, because this field is growing by leaps and bounds.

Read that small print!

It's true that the Federal government has not as yet set standards as to the definition of the term "low-calorie." So a manufacturer can label a product "low-calorie" even if it isn't, and still be in the clear. Read that small print, and be your own FBI.

In my favorite supermarket the other day, I saw in the dietetic food section a jar of expensive mayonnaise, labeled LOW-CALORIE. But the fine print stated that one teaspoon contained 33 calories. Now, if you know your calories, you know that regular mayonnaise is only 31 calories per teaspoon. Further along the shelf I saw DIET DELIGHT WHIPPED DRESSING, with a calorie count of only 8 calories per teaspoon. LOW-MAY is equally low-calorie.

Keep your calorie counter handy

I also admired a most attractive display of cookies, all labeled, largely LOW-CALORIE. But when I read the fine print, I found, for example, that on the box of vanilla wafers, the count per cookie was 34 calories; the 4-ounce package was expensive. Your old friends, the National Biscuit Company, have been putting out vanilla wafers for umpteen years. As your little calorie counter will tell you, each vanilla wafer contains only 20 calories. And a 3¾-ounce package of vanilla wafers was priced, in my market, at almost ⅓ the cost of the dietetic brand.

Most de-calorized foods are finds!

However, I have found few instances of chicanery. More and more of the new de-calorized packaged foods are reasonable in price, honestly trimmed away down in calories, and really delicious.

Tasti-Diet's sweet purple prune-plums, for example, are as good or better than any regular fruits in sugar syrup. The Diet-Sweet Elberta peach halves can't be beat—even by home-canned. They're big, shaggy, firm of fiber, and only 37 calories per 100 grams, instead of the 106 calories for the same amount of regular canned peaches.

Dietitian brand CHOC-LOW is as thick and fudgy a chocolate as you ever drizzled over ice cream, and only 5 calories in a teaspoon of it, versus 42 calories for ordinary chocolate syrup. I've never had a store-bought chocolate sauce that matches this thick, fluffy, creamy CHOC-LOW.

Almost anything can happen!

Such advances have been made just in the last year or so at removing calories without removing flavor, that almost anything delightful can happen in this direction. Consider some of these changes: from the pallid water-packed fruits, to the thick, new Sucaryl-sweetened syrups; from the thick wooden-tasting diet toasts and rusks, to the whole elegant new line of Devonshire melbas, Slim Krisp Melba, only 9 calories a slice, their Cheese Niblets, 1 calorie each: Wafer-ettes.

Because they're more expensive than regular foods, watch out when shopping in dietetic food sections and health stores for products labeled SALT-FREE. Not that there's anything wrong with them, except that they're often *not* low-calorie, and obviously they're going to taste pretty flat, without salt. There's no virtue in salt-free products for reducers; they won't reduce you. In fact, it is unwise to restrict your salt intake unless you've been advised to do so by your doctor for a specific condition. Except during very hot weather, when you need extra salt, you can allow your taste to be your guide as to the amount of salt you use in food.

Shop in the health food stores, too

There are still certain products you're going to have to shop for in health food stores. You'll find a dizzying assortment of teas, honeys, laxative products, and things labeled Low-Cholesterol, High-Carbohydrate, Low-Carbohydrate, Low-Sodium, High-Protein, Fortified, Salt-Restricted, Raw, Natural, Whole, Unrefined, and other confusing things. Keep calm and look for the calorie count of the contents on the label. If it isn't there, you can be sure it's because it's not low enough to be a selling point. Most low-calories fruits in health stores are the water-packed kind rather than the new Sucaryl-sweetened variety. Now you may like these juice-packed or water-packed fruits, and may prefer to do your own Sucaryl sweetening at home, since tastes differ. But read the label, and know what you're getting, at any rate.

Buy economy sized Sucaryl

A 1,000-tablet bottle of Sucaryl is the equivalent of over ten pounds of sugar; it costs least when you buy it this way. So does the liquid if you buy the 20-ounce bottle.

CHECK LIST OF DE-CALORIZED PACKAGED FOODS

Canned fruits

De-calorized by 30 per cent to 70 per cent in thick, sweet flavorful syrups which contain no sugar.

Because desserts are so often the Waterloo of reducers, these fruits are number one on your shopping list.

Use them in dozens of dessert recipes, from upside-down cakes to fruit jellos, from peach melba to applesauce cake, in compotes, in fruit cobblers, in shortcakes, and melon baskets. Use these fruits, too, in cocktails and fruit salads; as a side dish for meats.

Keep a can or two always in your refrigerator, and your supply cupboard well stocked with these wizard figure-savers. Order your favorites by the case and you'll save pennies as well as pounds. Because these de-calorized fruits are as inexpensive as any other dessert, and so much less fattening than almost anything you can serve, don't spare on your outlay for them.

	Calories (per 100 grams) De-calorized	Calories (per 100 grams) Regular fruits in heavy sugar syrup
Apricots	37	87
Pears	36	77

	Calories (per 100 grams) De-calorized	Calories (per 100 grams) Regular fruits in heavy sugar syrup
Cling Peaches, Halves and Slices	34	81
Elberta Peaches, Halves and Slices	37	106
Fruit Cocktail	38	78
Greengage Plums	36	110
Thompson Seedless Grapes	57	90
Kadota Figs	56	147
Prune-Plums	35	108
Dole Dietetic Pineapple	59	86

NOTE: In reading the ingredients listed on the labels of canned fruits in dietetic food sections, realize that cyclamate means Sucaryl. Sorbital contains as many calories as sugar, though they're more slowly absorbed.

Puddings

Butterscotch pudding, chocolate pudding, vanilla pudding, French custard, lemon pudding.

These de-calorized instant puddings are just as easy to make as the regular brands. Their taste and texture is the same; perhaps a trifle less sweet, which many people prefer. But you can always sweeten them more with Sucaryl, with tablets dissolved in the hot liquid you use in whisking them together.

They're de-calorized practically down to zero, as far as the dry mix itself goes. You can make them successfully with skimmed milk. There's almost no difference between the taste of skimmed and whole milk in these recipes. A half-cup serving made with skimmed milk is under 40 calories versus 140 calories for the regular puddings, even when made with skimmed milk.

Don't forget dress-up toppings. Chopped nuts, a dollop of whipped cream from an aerosol can, shredded coconut, a bit of crushed peanut brittle; and on the lemon pudding, a sprinkle of pulverized candy mints; all these add texture interest, as well as a luxurious look.

Don't forget how you can use these delicious de-calorized puddings in desserts: trifle, éclair fillings, cream pie fillings, as a base in fruit tarts and pies, cake fillings, crème brûlée (put a topping of brown sugar under the broiler till it browns and bubbles), blanc-mange, as a sauce on apple or peach scallop, Boston cream pie, mixed with ice cream or fruits, in a parfait glass, as a sauce on fresh or canned fruit.

Do keep a good supply of all pudding flavors on hand always, right in the front of your supply cupboard. They cost more than the regular kind but they help so wonderfully to keep the dessert calorie count down, they're worth their price. You'll find them in the dietetic food section of any supermarket.

Gelatin Desserts

De-calorized from 80 calories a serving to 10 *calories!*

For my money regular Jell-o isn't such a great low-calorie dessert; and pretty cheerless. But there are two ways you can de-calorize gelatin desserts; then you can serve nice big helpings and have them rich with fruit and nuts and whipped cream; for less calories than a tiny dish of the regular kind, bare and plain.

Method one: Start with Knox's plain gelatin, and use de-calorized fruit juices or the syrup from your de-calorized canned fruits. This broadens your repertoire, since it permits you to make these flavors: apricot, grapefruit, pineapple, grape, peach, prune-plum (which makes a really wonderful fruit Jell-o ring).

Method two: You can buy de-calorized gelatin desserts in these flavors: cherry, strawberry, raspberry, orange, lemon, and lime. Easy directions on the package are the same as for making Jell-o. The calorie count: per half-cup serving, 10 calories instead of 81.

If your reducers like Jell-o, these calories are worth saving, because you can serve gelatin desserts often, and give them seconds! Make sure your supply of this quick, easy, favorite dessert is never low. You'll add very few calories by adding your canned low-calorie fruits.

Look in your cookbook for gelatin dessert variations, sherbets, whips, and snows. For salads and aspics use this de-calorized Jell-o just as you would the regular kind.

Don't forget to use your fancy molds, and the dress-up toppings that take it out of the humdrum and into the de luxe category. Whipped cream, dusted with a grating of orange rind, is one elegant topping.

Fall Fruit Soufflé Salad

1 package lime or lemon D-Zerta
1 cup hot water
½ cup cold water
2 tablespoons lemon juice
½ cup Low-May
¼ teaspoon salt
1 cup diced, peeled apples
¾ cup seeded red grapes
¼ cup chopped walnuts

Dissolve D-Zerta in *hot water*. Add cold water, Low-May, lemon juice, and salt. Blend well with rotary beater. Pour into refrigerator freezing tray. Quick-chill in freezing unit (without changing control) 15 to 20 minutes, or until firm about 1 inch from edge but soft in center. Turn mixture into bowl and whip with rotary beater until fluffy. Fold in apples, grapes, walnuts. Pour into 1-quart or individual molds. Chill until firm in refrigerator (*not* freezing unit) 30 to 60 minutes. Unmold. Serves 4 to 6.

Ice-Cream Mixes

Dietitian Ice-Cream Mix has no calorie content at all. But it turns out that while the dry powder mix itself is saccharin-sweetened and innocent of calories, the recipe on the box calls for 1 cup of light cream! This contains approximately 500 calories. Since low-calorie store-bought ice cream contains only about 525 calories per pint, why bother?

Ice-Milk

A near-twin to ice cream in taste and texture. It comes in vanilla or a chocolate-strawberry-vanilla mix. Calorie-saving: about 25 per cent . . . worth-while, if you eat a lot of ice cream.

De-Calorized Candies and Cookies

You will find a variety of de-calorized candies and cookies, some of them looking very appetizing, in supermarkets and department stores. The widest assortment is likely to be found in a big up-to-date health food store. If you eat a good deal of candy and adore cookies, I would suggest that you try any and all of them that appeal to you.

I am not going to recommend any particular ones because I have found such a wide variance of preference among friends, acquaintances, and diet-book authors. I don't happen to like any of them very much, which is nice for me because these de-calorized candies and cookies are comparatively expensive. However, my daughter likes a lot of them; so do other people, and so may you.

Best buy: no-calorie sugarless hard candies. They're sweet and pleasant-tasting and come in every imaginable flavor: butterscotch, coffee, mint, molasses, licorice, wild cherry, honey, lemon, orange, toffee, all the fruit flavors. There are sugarless lollypops too. Some have almost no food value. Many are only a calorie or so each. This is considerably less than even the 15 or 20 calories ordinary hard candies contain. To a big candy eater, calorie savings on these sugarless hard candies will mount up importantly, over days and weeks and months.

More de-calorized candies to explore: chocolate mints, chocolate bars and squares, chocolate creme bars, orange, rum, mocha, or mint "party pieces," bonbons, chocolate-covered marshmallows, cat's tongues, coconut candies, assorted chocolates, soft fruity jells, chocolate-covered peppermint creme bars.

Some de-calorized cookies: coconut cookies, chocolate chippies, snaps (such as lemon, vanilla, chocolate, or ginger), creme-filled wafer sandwiches, fruit-tea cookies, lady fingers, sponge cookies, teatime cookies, almond crisps, petit fours, an assortment of party cookies called Teestays.

NOTE: Look for the calorie count per piece on the box. *If it isn't given, it isn't low.*

Candies made with honey and molasses, cookies made with whole-grain flours may be more wholesome but they're not likely to be any lower in calorie count. That's why you don't see the calorie count displayed anywhere. Consider, too, the size of the pieces. Could their tiny size account for the low-calorie count? You're paying a premium price for de-calorized goods, so read the label and make sure they're really de-calorized.

De-calorized beverages

Sugarless beverage concentrates: Kola, ginger ale, strawberry, root beer, raspberry, cherry, ginger are available. Add seltzer or club soda to a few teaspoons of the concentrate. Calorie count comes under 10 calories per drink.

Flav-R Straws, Fizzies: The first are straws with no-calorie flavor built in. At all markets. *Fizzies* are new flavor "cartridges which carbonate plain water."

Fruit juices: To my mind the best of these are Sucaryl-sweetened and made by the same companies who make the excellent canned fruits in Sucaryl-sweetened syrup: Pratt-Low's Diet-Sweet brand; Tillie Lewis's Tasti-Diet; Richmond Chase's Diet Delight.

You'll find almost every known variety of fruit juice canned without added sugar, salt, or water; and therefore low-calorie, but not very sweet. You may like them as is; or you can sweeten them to taste with saccharin or Sucaryl.

Nonfat Dry Milk: Big improvements here. Now, there's no foaming, no shaking, no lumping, no caking. It mixes in cold water (even in ice water) in seconds. All you need for the job is water, and a glass. And, as you know, this easy, economical, low-calorie milk has all the nutrients whole milk provides, except the fat.

Hot Chocolate: Dietitian Cocoa is made like any other cocoa: 17 calories in a heaping teaspoon of the dry mix. The calories, of course, are in the skimmed milk. I prefer to make cocoa with Choc-Low; the syrup mixes more easily, and has more of a chocolate flavor, to my mind.

De-Calorized Carbonated Soft Drinks: Do you remember to jazz those life savers up now and then with a slice of orange, a dash of lemon or lime, a few drops of sherry or liqueur, or a stick of cinnamon? Do you use them to make fruit desserts more interesting? Float melon balls in minted No-Cal Ginger Ale? Spark up blueberries with Cott's Raspberry Soda?

Chewing gums

In the dietetic food sections and food stores, you'll find sugarless chewing gums, in peppermint, spearmint, tropical fruit, and half a dozen other flavors as well as ammoniated sugarless gums. Your dentist may already have suggested these for yourself or your youngsters.

Some children like the distinction of being given a special kind of gum that won't hurt teeth. If you get this kind of a reaction, all well and good. It makes the dental reason-why for all the new sugarless foods and soft drinks seem consistent and believable. The actual calorie saving on gum is negligible, since ordinary gum contains only 1 to 5 calories per stick.

Phantom syrups, jams and jellies

Make your own phantom syrup by extending the maple-flavored Basic Sundae Sauce on page 113 with water. With real syrup costing 50 calories a tablespoon, it's worth while! Tillie Lewis makes a pancake syrup and a maple flavored syrup. (See page 44 for her address.)

Of course these phantom syrups aren't as good as the real thing. But a judicious mixture of these *and* the real thing is better than table syrups and

saves you plenty of calories. So, in a real maple syrup
bottle, combine one part real maple syrup to three parts
or more of the phantom syrup. The consistency will
be thinner, but the taste will be sweet and good and
fragrantly maple. A kind deed for waffle and pancake
lovers!

Sugarless Chocolate Syrups: Tillie Lewis's chocolate flavored topping has 8 calories in one tablespoonful. Write for it. The address: Tillie Lewis Foods,
Stockton, California 95201.

If your family likes chocolate, you should buy
Choc-Low by the case, and save money. Because
there's no end to the uses for it. Use it in beverages,
hot and cold; for sundaes, sodas, parfaits, fillings,
frostings, sauces, ice-box puddings, soufflés; in pies,
cakes, cookies. Choc-Low contains a mere 5 calories
per teaspoonful. It's so thick it will scarcely pour: a
richly dark chocolate color, and properly bittersweet.
(It's easy to add no-calorie sweetening when you want
a sweeter chocolate, and as is, it makes a fine taste
contrast to sweet bases, such as ice cream, cake, etc.)
It's not expensive either.

Sugarless Fruit Syrups (almost no-calorie): You
can use the better fruit drink concentrates as sundae
syrups, you will find. I liven them up a bit by adding
fruit flavors (see page 112) and sometimes Sweeta.
Also, a dash of lemon juice which seems to intensify
all fruit flavors. For thickness, mix them with a sugarless jam or jelly of the same flavor. Dietitian Strawberry Flavor Soda Mix has a syrup consistency, for
instance, and can be further thickened with a sugarless
strawberry jelly.

Sugarless Jams and Jellies: Three calories per teaspoon versus about 20 calories for sugar-sweetened
ones. Raspberry, strawberry, pineapple, orange, cherry,
grape, apricot, plum, apricot-pineapple,* and other
combinations. Some of these are woefully thin and
pale tasting. But improvements are rapidly being made
—so keep buying and trying new ones.

---

*Tasti-Diet is remarkably good!

Diet Sweet recently came out with half a dozen flavors; interesting, fresh-tasting, and a reasonable facsimile of the sugar-sweetened jams and jellies. Stir in a few chopped nuts for a texture dress-up. To sugarless raspberry jam add a teaspoon of the seediest kind of store-bought raspberry jam for verisimilitude. Another variation I like, is to add a few drops of sherry or the fruit brandy that "matches" the fruit flavor of the jam.

When you use jam or jelly on toast or waffles or muffins, cut down or skip butter altogether. Keep an assortment of these sweet fruit spreads on the table in attractive jam pots. If they're there, your weight-watchers will often use them instead of butter; or with cottage cheese; or perhaps with that wholesome yogurt, as a meal-finisher. These sugarless jellies help enormously in their humble way to keep those sweet teeth from aching.

De-calorized salad dressings
Up to 98 per cent less calories.

There are a lot of these; both mayonnaise-type dressings, and different French dressings. They're improving all the time. The texture's right; *you* add tartness and taste. (See p. 103–5.)

CAUTION: Look for the calorie count on the jar! You'll see some salad dressings in the dietetic food sections that are there because they're salt free, and not because they're de-calorized. There's considerable difference in the calorie content of those labeled low-calorie, too.

Only two sugarless sweeteners
Reducers' stand-by.

You'll see a dozen trade names, but, as of this writing all brand-name sweeteners are built either of Sucaryl or saccharin. The fine print on the label will tell you which; and identify a new no-calorie sweetener if and when one comes along. In cold drinks or uncooked dishes, one's as good as the other. Saccharin is supposed to be more concentrated. It costs a bit less than Sucaryl and dissolves a bit more readily. When cooking is required, Sucaryl is preferable. Saccharin seems to leave a slight bitter aftertaste.

To repeat what was said above, Sucaryl comes in three forms: 1. Sucaryl tablets (cyclamate sodium; the cheapest form) for use in drinks and recipes; 1 tablet has the sweetening power of 1 teaspoon of sugar. 2. Sucaryl sweetening powder, which comes in a convenient little bottle with a shaker top, so that you can dust Sucaryl on your fruit or cereal straight from the bottle. 3. Liquid Sucaryls. One of these two liquid forms of Sucaryl is required for people with low-sodium diets. You ask for calcium cyclamate. You can make up a supply of your own liquid Sucaryl (see p. 10).

Saccharin is sold under a multiple of trade names. True Sucaryl says "sodium cyclamate" in small type. But until we can get it again, it says only "saccharin" alas! You can buy saccharin in tablets, powder, crystals, or liquid form under a variety of trade names: Saxin, Sweet-Tabs, Sweet'N it, Sweeta, etc.

Miscellaneous

You'll find a couple of brands of peanut butter in the dietetic food sections. But don't get your hopes up! They're just as high-calorie as the regular brands; around 600 calories per 100 grams. "No salt or sugar added," you'll read on the label. But alas, it isn't salt or sugar that puts calories in peanut butter. It's peanuts.

Low-calorie peanuts exist, though. Look for them in your supermarket. They're less fattening because they're de-oiled. Only 17 calories in a handful instead of about 84! De-oiled—they're lighter in color, milder, and sweeter—but *just* as crisp and still mighty good eating! De-calorized peanut butter will be along soon too; look for it.

Products made of artichoke flour contain just about as many calories as those made of grain flours;

and don't let anybody tell you different. The rusks and breadsticks and noodles are very good, though.

The canned tuna fish in the dietetic section gives you a calorie saving of almost 40 per cent: 76 calories less in every serving. You'll find salmon in the dietetic food sections, too, but if you compare the calorie value with regular salmon in your calorie counter, you'll see that the calorie saving is negligible.

Moral: Always Read the Calorie Value on the Can! Compare it with your calorie tally.

Dorset have put out some canned main-course dishes such as beef stew, chicken fricassee, chicken with rice or vegetables, but these are prepared for salt-restricted diets and offer no worth-while calorie savings to reducers. There's no calorie saving on their Diet Pack Pea Soup, and yet their Diet Pack Tomato Soup is an excellent calorie buy. And their Cream of Mushroom Soup (made without sugar or salt) contains only 44 calories to a serving as against 180 for regular cream of mushroom soup. (Dilute with water. If you use skimmed milk, it comes to 77 calories per serving.)

See the check list of low-calorie staples on page 128. It's one I made in the course of a tour of a Grand Union supermarket in my neighborhood. These are not "dietetic" foods. You'll find different brand names in your part of the country, perhaps. And you'll be able to add to this list, as you shop in department stores and fancy food shops in your town.

Do add to this list. Add on the basis of your family's food favorites!

Take the list with you when you set out to stock up. Keep it by your telephone and check it as you do your daily ordering. Revise your shopping to eliminate foods that are supercharged with calories. This is the first step in the new twentieth-century lightweight cooking technology.

5

Low-protein Diet, or High—Which?

The vital role of protein has been unwittingly dramatized by the official protests of the Rockefeller Institute for Medical Research over the careless exploitation of diets originally designed by their Dr. Vincent P. Dole and his colleagues to aid in metabolic studies on human beings.

One of their major objectives in developing the Formula Diet was to achieve *maximum uniformity of intake,* a balanced diet that was easy for the Institute doctors to control, hard for the patients to cheat on. At one stage of the experiment, intake was reduced to 900 calories a day for a considerable period of time, which naturally caused loss of weight. (During this stage, a colloid preparation was occasionally found necessary to supplement the formula's lack of bulk, since the entire day's intake consisted of 2½ cups of liquid: a mixture of corn oil, water and dextrose.)

Evidence that the low-protein Formula Diet took off the pounds faster or satisfied hunger better than a high-protein diet—or any other diet—was never claimed by the Rockefeller Institute.

Another small study (thirty-two patients, ten outpatients) was aimed at discovering whether if the protein is limited, the patient will make it up in other foods. Results indicate that, to quote the Rockefeller Institute's report in the *American Journal of Clinical*

48

Nutrition, "a limitation of protein appears to be a useful adjunct in the treatment of obesity." A limitation of almost anything might be "a useful adjunct" in the treatment of obesity. (This conservative group doesn't even say *successful* treatment" of obesity!) Not much basis for the great hurra-burra going on about low-protein diets, is it?

According to *Time Magazine*'s Medical editor: "The 'Fabulous Formula' is essentially the same as a diet designed to produce liver disease and hardening of the arteries in laboratory animals." (*Time,* August 6, 1956)

Now this may well be an exaggeratedly pessimistic view as to the desirability of the low-protein diets —just as exaggerated as the hopped-up claims being made for their success.

Nevertheless, to date, the overwhelming weight of evidence from university, clinic and hospital research seems very much on the high-protein side.

But the more I read about nutrition and the more doctors I talk to about it, the more I am aware that the only *certainty* in our present state of knowledge is that of *change*. It's an area still chock-full of mythology and unsolved mysteries. No authority on nutrition is so august that there isn't an equally august one taking a directly opposite point of view! Or so it seems!

6

The Sex-Appeal Sixteen

Sixty-five or more nutrients are needed to keep you sleek, bright and full of life. They're as interdependent as the parts of an engine. You need them all. How they work together and the wonder each of them is capable of performing is the subject of a lot of other books. One of the most readable is the classic by Adele Davis and is called *Let's Eat Right to Keep Fit*.

It's a real thriller about nutrition—amusing, amazing, and as personal to *you* as your birth certificate.

The problem we're considering in this book, however, is how you can get these nutrients and still keep your daily calorie count down. Only when you know something about them can you spend calories cleverly to get the most life and looks and eating pleasure for every calorie.

You have often read that proteins are largely what make our body machine tick. The more high-quality protein you eat, the greater your sex appeal, the better your posture, muscle tone, hair, nails, skin, resistance to disease, digestion, and elimination. Your skin is largely *made* of the protein you eat. So is your hair and your brain. So are your eyes.

You get a whole new deal every six months; every 180 days sees a turnover of the protein you're made of. It follows that, if you've been taking in lots of high-quality protein for six months, you'll be a better-looking specimen, have a fresher, younger-looking skin; livelier hair; brighter, sharper eyes; springier muscles that can hold your bones in better posture.

But if you've been shortchanging your body on protein, I'm told you'll age faster in looks as well as in outlook on life. Your body can't manufacture a first-class specimen out of inadequate material. Each organ must be robbed to make the supply go around. Your skin, hair, nails, and bones may dry and thin; your muscles may lose tone; your energy and even your thinking can lack resilience.

It seems that the *kinds* of calories you eat are just as important as the number. Protein calories appear to be therapeutic and cosmetic calories, active nutrients that keep you young and elastic.

It's EXCESS *Protein that Speeds Slimming.* If you can take in twenty or thirty per cent more grams of protein per day than your body uses for rebuilding and repair, that excess protein will speed up weight reduction—provided, of course, that you haven't also taken in more calories than your body will use that day.

The Fewer Proteins, the More Water-Weight. Reducers, please note: even a mild protein deficiency causes a faulty elimination of waste-laden liquids from the body tissues. People who look fat are sometimes merely waterlogged.

A high protein intake performs other miracles for overweight people.

Excess protein tends to raise the metabolism, or the rate at which the body burns all its food fuel and stored fat.

It raises and upholds the blood sugar level. (Protein, not sugar, is the major factor here, contrary to what you may read in the advertisements. True, sugar raises the blood sugar level in minutes, but then it drops almost as fast.) On a low-calorie, high-protein

breakfast a reducer's spirits, energy, and efficiency get
a pickup that is sustained up to six hours.

The craving for sweets tends to disappear when
the blood sugar level is kept high. (Reduces your
dentist bill as well as your waistband!)

The experience of most people checks with most
clinical tests, which indicates that proteins not only
satisfy your appetite faster, but they keep it satisfied
longer; you seem to get less hungry between big protein
meals . . . "They stick to your ribs," you say.

How much protein do you need?

You may use the following rule for gauging an
adult's individual protein needs per day: for each
pound of your "ideal" weight, ½ gram of protein. So, if
the right weight for you is 140 pounds, your minimum
daily requirement is 70 grams of protein.

How much have you been getting? Use food tables and try to figure it out. It's vital that you keep
track or chances are you won't get enough.

The high-quality proteins most people know
about are expensive—eggs, steaks, chops, roasts. People with low incomes almost invariably suffer from
protein deficiency. But surveys show that 60 per cent
of the people who have money to eat anything they
choose, also get far less protein than they need.

Here's a list of sixteen sex-appeal foods you
should know by heart. All are good calorie buys. Yes,
the nuts and peanut butter are high-calorie but they're
also unusually high in vitamins and/or minerals as
well as two rare, essential fatty acids. You use them in
small quantities. And remember their psychological importance in making a reducer feel he's eating luxuri-
ously, not being deprived of good things.

There are, of course, many other foods not listed
here which supply protein, but most of these either
contain incomplete proteins or contain more calories,
too. NOTE: an "incomplete" protein is lacking in two
or more of the twenty-two known amino acids of which
a "complete" protein is composed. All twenty-two are
vital to health.

The Sex-Appeal Sixteen

Foods (100 grams) Approx. 3½ ounces	Calories	Grams Protein	For Quick Tally Approx. No. Calories per Protein Gram
Beef			
Chipped	203	34.3	6
rib roast	319	24	13
sirloin	297	23	13
porterhouse	185	26.4	7
corned, lean	263	23.5	10
round steak	233	27	8
Cottage Cheese	108	20	5
Cheese (average	370	20	18
Cheddar	398	25	16
Parmesan	393	36	11
Swiss	370	27.5	13
Egg	162	12.8	12
Fish			
bluefish	124	20.5	5
flounder	65	14.9	4
haddock	79	18.2	4
mackerel	223	17.4	10
cod, fresh	74	16.5	5
cod, dried	375	81.8	5
crab meat	104	16.9	6
clams	81	13	6
lobster	88	16.2	5
shrimps	127	26.8	5
oysters	84	9.8	8
sardines	214	25.7	8
tuna fish	198	29	6
halibut	179	18.6	6
Fowl			
chicken, breast of	104	23.3	4
chicken, dark meat	112	20.5	4
turkey	268	20.1	13
Lamb, lean	235	18	18

Foods (100 grams) Approx. 3½ ounces	Calories	Grams Protein	For Quick Tally Approx. No. Calories per Protein Gram
Milk			
skimmed, dry, solids	362	35.6	10
liquid skimmed milk			
(1 cup, 246 grams)	87	8.6	10
buttermilk			
(1 cup, 244 grams)	86	8.5	10
whole milk			
(1 cup, 244 grams	168	8.5	20
Nuts			
almonds	597	19	31
peanuts	559	26.9	20
Organ meats			
liver	140	20	7
heart	108	16.9	6
tongue	207	16.4	11
kidneys	114	16.3	9
Peanut Butter	576	26.1	212
Pork, lean; ham	312	22.8	13
Vienna sausage	215	15.8	13
Canadian bacon	231	22.1	10
Soybean flour	228	44.7	5
Veal, lean	164	19.71	8
Wheat germ	361	25.2	14
Yeast, brewer's, pow- dered	273	36.9	7

The Big Four

To sum up: of all proteins available, the most nutrient-loaded, the most concentrated, low-calorie, and least expensive, are brewer's yeast, cottage cheese, wheat germ, and powdered skimmed milk. Cottage cheese is a "natural"; delicious, easy, versatile. See page 59.

These *Big Four* can go right down your gullet, straight, with no calories added in mixings.

Low-fat soy flour is equally valuable, and low cost too. But it takes cooking time and added calories to transform it into baked goods. And the unfamiliar taste presents a problem in making them welcome at a conservative eater's table.

Yeast, being loaded with B vitamins, gives you an appetite. So skip it when you go on a two-day diet treat (see page 164) designed to shuffle off quickly three or four pounds that have crept up on you when you weren't looking. You need all the low-calorie protein you can get when you're on a get-thin-quick diet treat, but fortunately you can get it without a built-in appetite inducer.

Four more stand-outs for potency

Notice what a whacking big lot of protein you get for your calories in dried beef, the least expensive form of beef you can buy! 34.3 grams for 203 calories—the best protein calorie buy among all meats, including the most expensive. Good with scrambled eggs, good in corn pudding, good creamed; good with cottage cheese in nice thick sandwiches. Remind yourself to explore for new ways to serve it. And have it *oftener*.

Round steak a close second. Note how fast fish can slim you, build youthful bounce and good looks, too.

Organ meats also deserve to be starred often in your menus for their low cost, low calorie, high protein. And you're justified in serving chicken as often as you'd like; buy the breasts in a "parts" store and feast on them.

7

Eat Your Milk

The dictum that everybody needs to drink at least a quart of milk a day is one of those oversimplified rule-of-thumb pronouncements meant for people assumed to be nutritionally illiterate.

The mother who unquestioningly accepts this idea has very little chance of getting her child's weight down.

Half the calories in whole milk are butterfat. Instead of drinking them, *un*consciously, have the conscious pleasure of eating what butter calories you do decide to take in.

Problem: how to get the calcium without calories?

Now, it's true that everybody needs the calcium that's packed into milk products in greater quantity than in any other food. Milk products are the only dependable source of calcium in our diet. The only low-calorie source of calcium is skimmed milk products—nonfat dry milk, buttermilk, and easiest of all, fresh cottage cheese.

Children, pregnant and nursing mothers, old people, need more calcium and need it more critically than the rest of us—but to all of us, it's a staff of life that bread never was.

Public health authorities say that a calcium deficiency is the commonest of all our nutrient deficiencies; it's right up there along with not getting enough

56

protein. What are the typical symptoms of a calcium deficiency? Nervous tension. Inability ro relax. Susceptibility to nervous fatigue.

How calcium relates to overweight

Here are three good reasons why people put on extra pounds. When fat-prone people who are chronically tense approach the cocktail hour, their defenses are down. Because their nervous fatigue is greater, they need more drinks to pick them up. They tend to drink them faster than other people, because all their motions are speeded up, including the hand-to-mouth motions with the potato chips, the salted nuts, and the canapés.

It's tenseness, inability to relax, as much as childhood conditioning, that's behind the terrifically fattening habit of bolting one's food; taking big mouthfuls, eating fast, swallowing fast, washing food down with quick mouthfuls of whatever there is to drink, and therefore eating more.

Insomnia, the nighttime manifestation of inability to relax, is one of the symptoms of a calcium deficiency. There are health, business, and cosmetic reasons for getting over insomnia. Also there's the tendency to get up for a drink and a soothing snack during those wakeful, worried hours.

Do you know how much calcium you need? Here's a jingle to help you remember:

A gram of calcium a day
Will help you weigh what you *want* to weigh!

Yes, you need one full gram—1000 milligrams —of calcium a day. Fortunately your body stores it, so you can store up in advance against what medical books call "times of dietary insult."

If you're calcium-starved, drinking even two quarts of milk a day wouldn't catch you up. And even if you aren't, it takes careful meal planning to get in a daily gram of calcium and keep the calorie count down, even using skimmed-milk products.

Eat your milk the no-calorie way

There's a way to get calcium without calories, as a food supplement and calcium-insurance policy. Stock up on calcium lactate, either in tablet or powder form. Or fine bone powder: *not* bone meal or ground bone. Why so fussy about the form your calcium supplement takes? Because your body doesn't absorb calcium readily. The hydrochloric acid in your stomach will dissolve the powdered bone, but not the coarser ground bone.

Even the calcium in whole sweet milk isn't absorbed as readily as in yogurt (you can often use yogurt in place of sour cream), cultured buttermilk, and cottage cheese, because helpful lactic acid is present in these particular milk products.

Eat your milk in its highest-protein form

Protein is enormously helpful in increasing the absorption of calcium. So is that 1 to 2 tablespoons of unhydrogenated oil you should be getting every day in nuts salad oil, or fresh peanut butter.

Eat your milk in the form of cheese

Stock up on your pet cheeses to stop dieting and start losing. With a juicy apple, a hunk of your favorite cheese makes a filling, long-lasting, luxurious snack or dessert course.

For about the same number of calories as goes down in one quick glass of whole milk, look how much good solid eating you can enjoy!

> 6 big tablespoons of snowy, fresh-tasting cottage cheese or ricotta
> or 2 sandwich slices of Swiss cheese
> or 2 wedges of creamy Camembert, Gruyère, or Roquefort cheese
> or 3 tablespoonfuls of almost all the Kraft cheese spreads: olive, pimento, pineapple, etc.
> or a serving of fluffy, fragrant cheese soufflé
> or almost ¼ pound of solid, mild, smoky-tasting Provolone cheese.

Cottage cheese—reducer's "best buy"

You can eat cottage cheese till the cows come home and never gain weight. It's made of skimmed milk, with a little whole milk added in what's called "creamed" cottage cheese, delicate in flavor, fluffy, buttery smooth.

You'll tend to lose, not gain, on cottage cheese because it contains such a terrific charge of the highest quality protein. One of those 8-ounce containers of cottage cheese contains 44 grams of protein, 218 milligrams of calcium, and only about 215 calories. Now, a quart of whole milk only contains 34.2 grams of protein. You'd have to drink 2½ pints of regular milk (865 calories) to get as much protein as in that container of snowy fresh cottage cheese.

It's also one of the foods in which essential amino acids are supplied in great abundance. Cost: well under $2.00 for that 44 grams of Grade-A cottage cheese protein. Five rib lamb chops won't give you as much protein, will cost you 850 calories and heaven knows how much money.

Eat cottage cheese straight in a big whopping luncheon salad, with pineapple, peaches, apricots, melon. Eat it mixed with a spring salad of chives and crisp chopped red radishes. To lose weight and enjoy it, make a habit of these salads for lunch.

Easy, inexpensive, delicious

The low-fat brands of cottage cheese or pot cheese taste fine nowadays. These contain only 5 calories less per ounce than the regular creamed cottage cheese. Eat whichever you prefer—both are delicious.

Use cottage cheese in thick sandwich fillings; with chopped olives, pimento, chives, or minced radishes, or nuts, or jam. Children love it.

Use cottage cheese as a filling for fruit jello rings served as a salad, or as a dessert.

Fill a ripe cantaloupe with cottage cheese, either for a first course or dessert. These two flavors love each other.

Serve cottage cheese as a side dish with

chicken and cranberry sauce. Beat cottage cheese
in with your next tomato aspic. Wonderful!

Put cottage cheese on the table often in a
partitioned dish with other relishes: pickles, low-
calorie jams, etc. It's an especially good flavor
contrast with pickled beets or rosy cinnamon
apple rings.

Put half a cup of cottage cheese into your
next scrambled eggs, with or without chipped beef
and minced onion.

Salt and pepper cottage cheese and use it as
a sauce on vegetables such as asparagus, boiled
onions, broccoli. When cooked it melts into a
fluffy, stringy, cheesy mass.

Fill big green pepper halves with cottage
cheese; garnish with pimento or pineapple. Or
bake them (see recipe on page 94).

The golden, fluffy, delectable hollandaise
sauce recipe on page 21, is practically pure cottage cheese. Top fish, veal, chicken, vegetables
with it.

Put cottage cheese on the table for breakfast. This sounds strange, but it's good on toast
instead of butter. Load the de-calorized jam on
top!

Make low-calorie "sour cream" of cottage
cheese by whipping 1 cup of it in an electric
blender. If it's dryish, add ¼ cup water.

Get acquainted with farmer cheese

Find farmer cheese in a supermarket or Jewish
delicatessen. It comes in bulk or in a little package
like cream cheese.

It looks rather like cream cheese, tastes a bit like
cream cheese, has much the same suave texture, but is
less than a *fourth* as fattening as cream cheese. Lower
in price, too. Packed with protein and calcium, a
magnificent fat-fooler!

Experiment with it in any recipe in which you'd
use cream cheese; in frostings, in sandwich fillings,
cocktail spreads and dunks, in salad dressings, as a
dessert with low-calorie jam or jelly; whip it with a little
skimmed milk for a dessert-pancake filling (serve low-

calorie strawberry preserve topping over the warm pancakes).

Try the whipped cream cheeses, too. More air, fewer calories—and *heaven!*

How to save on butter calories

Butter calories mount up wickedly; this is the fattest food of all. Even a *little* butter is a lot of calories.

When you do serve butter, use whipped butter or better yet—margarine made of polyunsaturated oils. It's the fluffiest, freshest-tasting, most delectable kind of butter; and because it's partly air, it has about 30 per cent less calories per serving.

8

America's Favorite Recipes—
De-calorized

DRINK UP, EVERYBODY!

Question: Does drinking between meals make one fat?
Answer: Obviously, this depends largely on how many
calories lurk in your drink.

If it's water, soda water, or low-calorie soft drinks,
the answer is no.

We're about 90 per cent water; but the liquid
turnover of our body machines is very fast. Normally,
our water level stays pretty much the same. What largely determines the amount of water retained by the tissues is the amount of salt we take in. So don't oversalt
food. But, unless you *have* been oversalting food, you
won't achieve any permanent loss of weight by cutting
down on salt.

Drinking much with meals can act to make you
gain weight, but it's not just the calories in what you
drink that does the dirty work. It's also the fact that
people who "wash their food down" tend to eat *faster*
than other people, and therefore eat *more*.

Hints on how to wean overweights

Consistently "forget" to put anything to drink on
the table with meals.

If you *have* to produce a drink, make it as un-interesting as possible; water preferably. And not very cold water.

Bring it in a smallish water goblet rather than in a full 8-ounce tumbler. And don't quite *fill* even that smallish goblet.

Knowing your family as you do, you can devise other gambits which will wean them away from washing down their food. HEALTH NOTE: The juices furnished by the mouth and stomach do a better job in their digestive work when undiluted by water.

Do your drinking before you eat

Drinking a lot of something that's low-calorie and pleasant-tasting an hour or so before you eat can be a big factor in lowering your calorie intake—and your weight. A low-calorie liquid pause that refreshes will often delay, or eliminate entirely, a big fattening snack.

Let's see how this works. Suppose you've been shopping, happily, absorbedly, every faculty concentrated on the job. An hour or two passes. Then suddenly you realize that you're about ready to drop.

"Whew! I've got to stop for an ice-cream soda or something," you say to yourself. "Right this minute!"

Is it hunger you're feeling? If it's snack-time, but not meal-time, the chances are you're mostly thirsty. And tired.

Thirst is often mistaken for hunger

Yes, thirst is often mistaken for hunger. By children. By husbands. By you.

After dogging it intently about the stores awhile, you're tired all over. And you're dry all the way down to your stomach. Whether your stomach is empty or not, it knows darn well that it's unhappy. It wires an imperative message to your brain to that effect. At the same time your brain gets an SOS from your feet. Also from your parched mouth, and fagged musculature. It reacts to this pandemonium of messages with a quick but sloppy summary of this situation. The garbled translation that gets through to your consciousness goes something like this: "That all-gone feeling must mean you're hungry, you poor thing. Just relax now, Lovie, and give yourself a treat. You deserve it."

Actually what your body may want more than dry solid food is to feel a flood of pleasant-tasting wet stuff gurgling down your throat, refreshing your mouth, moistening your interior, restoring your juices. And you want to take the load off your feet.

If you do stop in at a soda fountain, chances are you'll order your ice-cream soda and then say, "But give me a big glass of water right away, please!" After the water you get the ice-cream soda. And you proceed to suck up 450 calories that you need like a broken arm.

But if you're hep to this particular mix-up of messages that the central nervous system is prone to, you'll ask for that big glass of water, quick, please; and then order tea or coffee and, say, a fruit cup, or cool juicy melon, or tart-sweet grapefruit—only about 50 calories instead of 450.

Water them first; feed them later

When your child comes ravening in from school, when your husband comes wiltedly home from work, whenever it's coming up for snack-time, morning, afternoon, or night, make this your rule: "Water" them first; feed them later. The whole trick is having long, delicious thirst-quenchers ready, waiting, on display.

(NOTE: For grownups, even if beer, or highballs, or cocktails are to follow, put your husband's favorite nonalcoholic thirst-quencher under his nose first. Let him tank up on the lowest-calorie liquids first, so that the calorie-rich alcoholic liquids won't have the bulk job of slaking his thirst. He'll drink less at the cocktail hour. Eat less at dinner, too.)

Summary: 5 reasons for drinking up

1. Thirst is often mistaken for hunger.
2. A definite-tasting drink often makes one's mouth change its mind about needing food.

3. A lot of definite-tasting drink often makes one's stomach change its mind about feeling empty. (Because then it isn't; at least for awhile.)
4. A thorough wetting, then a period of leisurely sipping keeps one's esophagus busy, damp, and pleasantly diverted.
5. Have "eating" fun, with festive, delectable, low-calorie drinks—because as a result one eats less, and therefore, loses faster.

Rule 1: Stage and produce the drink-making. If possible, fix a soft-drink "bar," complete with an electric mixer all attached, ready to flip on; and all the makings on display: vanilla, cinnamon stricks, bottles of liquid sweetener, jars of crystal-sweeteners, garnishes. Also, tall glasses, mugs, stirrers, tray, bottle openers, a full ice bucket.

Have a tea-tray set up all the time. All those generations of English can't be wrong.

Rule 2: Keep well-stocked with a variety of

(a) the new sugarless carbonated beverages, such as the new de-calorized ginger ale, black raspberry, black cherry, root beer, vanilla cream soda, lemon soda, orange soda, loganberry punch.

(b) Flav-R straws assorted fruit flavors (also chocolate). *So easy,* so pretty, so cheap to have a sweet no-calorie fruit drink. Just plop a few straws in the liquid, stir and sip! Sweetness and flavor flow magically from the straw into the water—and into you. I keep Flav-R straws in assorted flavors in a copper luster mug on the bar—a decorative and figure-saving bar accessory. If you find "Fizzies," keep them handy here too. Don't forget the new fruit juices, sweetened without sugar: chilled apple juice, apricot nectar, grape juice, grapefruit juice, pineapple juice. Also the low-calorie fruit concentrates, to which you may add water, tea, or soda water and dips of low-calorie ice cream, to a low-calorie ice-cream soda. (See page 112.)

Rule 3: Keep well-stocked with Sucaryl or saccharin in forms which dissolve in cold liquids as well as hot. For this, you can buy liquid saccharin such as Sweeta, or use liquid Sucaryl.

Rule 4: If your family is fond of chocolate drinks, be sure to keep a supply of sugarless chocolate syrup, or low-calorie prepared cocoa mix in plain sight, always.

Rule 5: For drinks which use milk, make an extra low-calorie skimmed milk with only *one* tablespoon of fat-free instant dry milk to 8 ounces of water. This amounts to only 25 calories, and when you've added coffee, cocoa, or sugarless chocolate syrup, and those aromatic flavorings, most thirsty people won't know the difference.

It wouldn't be hard to *drink* as many calories as you *eat* in one day. Overweight children can easily absorb 700 or 800 calories in a day between glasses of milk and bottles of assorted sweet soda pops. Grown-ups, also, without even being aware of it, are likely to drink 700 or 800 calories; milk, cocktails, highballs, a pop in the afternoon, a nightcap.

Traditional, unthinking drinking figures out at 80 to 300 calories per drink.

These de-calorized drinks are never over 60 calories per drink, and most of them are between 3 and 30 calories a drink. Result: Your daily calorie saving on drinks is likely to add up to 500 calories, if you modernize your drinking thinking as suggested in the following pages.

What'll you have?

A big pitcher of tea, hot or cold? Try different blends and fragrances—black Russian tea, jasmine tea.

Sweetened? (with Sucaryl)

With milk? (skimmed)

Dressed up? By all means! Clove-dotted lemon slicles, halved maraschino cherries. Fresh mint, when you can get it. Pineapple fingers. Whole fresh strawberries or a few blueberries.

A frosty cold pitcher of lemonade? De-calorized: 10 calories (traditional: 104 calories). Yes, thanks to Sucaryl, lemonade can be a great low-calorie refresher and pickup, cram-jammed with vitamin C, which is a specific to cure fatigue, especially summer fatigue. Don't forget the dress-ups: fresh mint, a handful of red raspberries, maraschino cherry halves.

Hot coffee? Iced coffee? An *ice-cold* low-calorie Kola drink; sugarless ginger ale; or other Sucaryl-sweetened bottled soft drinks? Practically every known flavor is now available in your supermarket.

WARNING: Don't discuss the fact that these are the dietetic variety of soft drinks any more than is necessary. You want your family to forget dieting, remember? Don't explain at all, unless you're asked.

MOTHERS, PLEASE NOTE! If, and when, you do have to explain or identify them, *tell your family that these sugarless drinks are better for everybody's teeth.* This is a generally accepted fact—an important *plus* Sucaryl has to offer. And as a reason for serving these wonderful new drinks, this explanation is more socially acceptable than their calorielessness.

Solid Drink Suggestions—the calorie count given is for 8 full ounces.

Frosted Coffee: 60 calories (traditional recipe: 300 calories). In electric mixer, combine 8 ounces of tepid coffee, 1 tablespoon of skimmed-milk powder, a few shakes of powdered Sucaryl or a few drops of Sweeta. Whip to a foamy froth.

Pour into a tall glass. Float 2 tablespoons of low-calorie vanilla ice cream on top.

Mexican Chocolate: 22 calories (traditional recipe: 265 calories). To each 8 ounces of hot water, add one envelope of low-calorie cocoa mix, and ¼ teaspoon ground cinnamon. Whip with electric mixer until frothy over low heat. Serve while still frothy with tall cinnamon stick in the mug or glass.

Milk Shakes: approximately 40 calories each 8-ounce serving (traditional recipes: 185 to 350 calories). For these use an electric blender. The procedure is the same for all. Place ½ cup of tepid water in the container. Add 1 tablespoon skimmed-milk powder, Sweeta to taste, chocolate or fruit (see below). Put on cover and turn on blender. Run for a minute. Add ½ cup of cracked ice to chill the shake and more Sweeta if desired. Put on cover and turn on blender; let it run for another minute. Pour into tall glass and serve.

CHOCOLATE: 2 tablespoons low-calorie chocolate syrup.
PEACH: ½ cup of fresh peaches.
STRAWBERRY: ½ cup fresh strawberries, 2 tablespoons juice.
APRICOT: ½ cup of fresh apricots, or 4 halves dietetic canned peaches, 2 tablespoons juice.
PINEAPPLE: ½ cup diced fresh pineapple.
RASPBERRY: ½ cup of fresh raspberries.
BANANA: ½ of a *small* banana, or ⅓ of a larger banana.
Make sure it's *rotten* ripe; the riper, the more flavor.

Hot Beef Bouillon or Hot Chicken Consommé: 1 serving (3 from 1 can), 27 calories. Very comforting on a cold day, midmorning, or midafternoon. If you use bouillon or consommé cubes dissolved in hot water, only 3 to 8 calories per cup, but not nearly as good, for my money.

Clam Juice, Tomato Juice or V-8: hot or cold, 50 calories for 8 ounces. Have a handful of cheese tidbits or oysterettes with it; only 1 calorie apiece.

CANAPÉS

There's a lot to be said for "spoiling" your appetite before dinner with low-calorie nibbles and a stomach full of liquids. Mothers of underweight children know how this before-meal stoking takes the edge off appetite, so why shouldn't it have the same effect on an overweight's appetite?

The interval between lunch and dinner is likely to be somewhat longer than between breakfast and lunch. If overweight is the problem, it's far better strategy to find long cool drinks, and a quick bite ready as the "patient" comes in the door, rather than to wait for dinner, getting hungrier, and probably crosser, by the minute. The trick, of course, is to keep these before-dinner bites so low in calories that even reasonably reckless nibbling can't add up to very many calories. (See Shopper's Check List on page 128—no-work ideas for your canapé shelf.)

And fortunately the kind of eating that goes with drinks, traditionally, includes so many low-calorie items that there's no need to fall back on the banal and murderously fattening potato chips and salted nuts.

With the family so hungry, whatever you have set out for them will be warmly welcomed, if you have made it look as appetizing as you know how. Every age enjoys the ease of eating with the fingers, too. So don't begrudge the time it takes to make a colorful bowl of crisp cold vegetables, or a big plate of pink shrimps, with a sauce; or "crackers" around several bowls of assorted creamy spreads.

This kind of family-spoiling is the kind of personal, loving attention that makes a woman mighty popular. And it works marvels at putting everybody in a cheerful, relaxed mood for dinner and a peasant evening together.

Canapés: First Principles

The key word for canapés is palate *titillation. So rule one is: keep coming up with new ideas.* Try new condiments, new combinations.

And remember to titillate the *eye,* as well as the palate. Make your canapé trays just as snobbish and festive, both in looks and character, as your talent allows. Creative canapé ideas get a hostess more kudos, cause more talk about her taste and originality—why is that, do you suppose?

Rule two: use low-calorie canapé bases. Instead of the usual crackers (16 to 24 calories each) use no-calorie canapé bases, or a cracker base that's only 5 calories. Suggestions for these follow.

Rule three: use low-calorie "cream" cheese base for spreads. Instead of butter (200 calories per ounce) or cream cheese (106 calories per ounce) use plain or whipped cottage cheese (around 24 calories per ounce). There's no end to the variety of spreads you can begin this way. Whip cottage cheese to whipped cream smoothness in your electric blender before adding seasonings. A supply of this in your refrigerator will keep for days. Suggestions follow.

Rule four: for moistening spreads, fillings, and bases, use ready-bought low-calorie French dressing or mayonnaise, at 1 to 24 calories per tablespoon instead of regular mayonnaise (92 calories per tablespoon); buttermilk, at 4 calories per tablespoon instead of cream (30 to 50 calories per tablespoon); low-calorie cream sauce (see basic recipe No. 1, page 14), at 3 calories per tablespoon, instead of the 50 to 70 calories per tablespoon in the traditional cream sauce recipe.

Rule five: concentrate on fish, lean meat, cottage cheese and other low-calorie ingredients, instead of fatty patés, salted nuts, fried and pastry-wrapped bundles. And don't spare the seasonings—fresh horseradish, curry, scallion tops, caraway seeds.

Rule six: make canapés and hors d'oeuvres small ones. It's flavor, it's variety, it's *titillation* you're dramatizing. That's what will make your canapés memorable and satisfying, rather than brute bulk.

Traditional canapés seldom contain less than 50 calories, and the majority of them are nearer 100 calories. None of the canapés suggested in the following pages is over 25 calories, and most of them are between 5 and 15 calories each. Result: a calorie saving on your bites-with-drinks every day, of 200 to 400 calories—and these de-calorized canapés are just as festive-looking, just as flavorful. And they'll leave you just as full—though definitely *not* as fattened.

Canapé Bases, approximately 5 calories each:

> Protein whole grain wafers. (Devonshire makes some. There's also a brand called Waferettes made by Hol-Grain Products Company.) Ideal Swedish Flat-bread. (Also a brand called Kavli Crispbread.) Melba toast rounds.

Canapé Bases, virtually no-calorie each:

> Sweet green or red pepper cut into rectangles, squares, or circles.
> Big mushroom caps, raw, broiled, or baked. Make a specialty of these, they're delicious, luxurious, *no*-calorie, and actually not expensive *per* mushroom cap.
> Celery stalks, in cut sections.
> Cucumber, sliced crosswise or lengthwise
> Zucchini, sliced crosswise or lengthwise

Canapé Spreads with no-calorie base, 5 calories per canapé—with 5-calorie base, 10 calories per canapé:

> *Clam Appetizer:* In electric blender whip together ½ pound cottage cheese or pot cheese with a 7½-ounce can minced clams, drained, ½ small onion, grated, one teaspoon Worcestershire, a dash

of garlic salt, and one teaspoon celery salt, plus
one teaspoon of the clam juice. Serve this spread
on melba toast rounds. Or heap it on mushroom
caps and put under the broiler a few minutes.
Or make a dip of it by adding more clam juice,
and serve it in a bowl, surrounded by raw cauliflower buds, to be dipped in it.

Curry "Cream" Cheese Spread: Start with 1 cup
of whipped cottage cheese. Season with salt, curry
powder, and caraway seeds for texture interest
as well as flavor.

Roquefort Spread: To 1 cup of whipped cottage
cheese, add Roquefort, and salt, to taste.

No-work Spreads: Put out trays of canapé bases;
in the center of the tray put a jar of one or
more of the following whipped cream cheese
spreads: olive-pimento; bacon-horseradish. Since
all of these are only about 60 to 70 calories per
heaping tablespoonful, a reasonable amount of
spread on a small canapé base will amount to
about a third of a teaspoonful or 7 to 10 calories
per dollop.

FAVORITE FIRST COURSES

How to out-think your stomach

Want to get fat fast? Don't have a first course.

Want to lose weight? Always have a first course.
If you want to lose weight fast, have a *couple* of first
courses, one of them being a salad.

This is the first principle of meal planning for
overweights: spoil the appetite and spare the pounds.

What's *hot* fools the stomach into thinking it's
getting more fodder than it is. A bowl of hot and
hearty beef soup will seem more filling to most men
than apple juice—but the beef soup contains far fewer
calories than the apple juice.

What's *sweet* has satiety value, and will take the
edge off an appetite nicely. Yet, half a big, ripe, sweet

cantaloupe contains a mere 50 calories! Half a broiled grapefruit, still bubbling, fragrant with sherry, combines hot with sweet. One hundred calories for this important-looking first course.

What's *big-scale* deceives the eye. Which would look like more to your man: a little glass of prune juice or a dozen clams spread out on the half shell with cocktail sauce? Same calorie cost! Don't forget artichokes, hot or cold.

Brute Bulk makes salad a good meal-opener. And since it's an essential *food,* it's essential to serve it *when it will be eaten.* Served before the main course salad will be enjoyed to the very last bite. Served after the main course, you'll so often find that it barely gets nibbled, that you wonder why you bother to make it.

A first course needn't mean a lot of extra work

Use a tray cart to serve each course from one big matriarchal dish: your big handsome soup tureen, your salad bowl, a casserole, a juice pitcher.

Extra bonus: Serving a stylish first course, and discovering good appetite-spoilers, will tend to get you out of that menu rut that lies in wait for all of us. You'll be as stimulated as your family, by the change.

Reminder List of First Course Favorites— all 100 calories or less per serving

Heinz Cream of Green Pea— only 73 calories per serving! Surprise!

(A serving of Campbell's contains 102 calories, it happens.) Pea soup is such a favorite with many men that I'll pause to suggest variations, typical of the ways you can add importance to consommés, bouillons, as well as pea soup.

Make it meaty: Add ½ cup of chopped tongue, salami, or any other cooked, lean meat.

Pennies from frankfurter: Float thin slices of frankfurter on top.

Special topping: A bit of grated sharp cheese and crumpled crisp bacon.

Curry twist: Mix ½ to 1 teaspoon of curry with ½ cup of cottage cheese and heat this with soup. Top with slivered almonds.

Sour cream float: Top each serving with a dollop of sour cream and chopped olives or scallions.

Mushroom hash: Add 1 cup chopped mushrooms when heating.

Parmesan toast float: Sprinkle melba toast rounds with Parmesan and warm under broiler. Float a round on each serving.

Other garnishes: Popcorn, chopped pimento, or ripe olives, garlic croutons, lemon slices, paprika, water cress, oysterettes, fried Chinese noodles, a mint leaf. And don't forget combinations of soup flavors; or adding a bit of sherry, or whatever wine is congenial to the soup you're serving.

SOUPS TO REMEMBER

Brand	Flavor	Calories per serving*
Campbell's	Beef	94
"	Beef Noodle	51
Heinz	Beef Noodle	68
"	Beef with Vegetables	62
Campbell's	Bouillon	27
"	Chicken Gumbo	49
Heinz	Chicken Noodle	71
"	Chicken Rice	36
"	Clam Chowder	70
"	Consommé	29
"	Gumbo Creole	65
Campbell's	Ox-tail	77
"	Pepper Pot	90
"	Scotch Broth	96
"	Vegetable	68
"	Vegetable-Beef	86
Heinz	Vegetable-Beef	81
"	Vegetable-no meat	81
Campbell's	Vegetarian vegetable	63
Dorset Diet-Pack	Cream of mushroom	44
Dorset Diet-Pack	Tomato	32

*Three servings from one can.

Soups are full of calorie surprises, aren't they? Why isn't cream of tomato soup here? It sounds low-calorie. But it's twice as fattening as beef noodle soup, which sounds like as hearty a soup as is going. Clear tomato soup contains only 84 calories a serving, *if* you can find it. I couldn't. Fortunately there's Dorset's fine Diet-Pack Tomato Soup. Stock up on it! Save more than 100 calories on every bowl you serve.

Cream of mushroom soup is such a favorite and so helpful for a quick sauce, that I was delighted to find that Dorset's Diet-Pack Cream of Mushroom comes well within a calorie counter's "budget"—only 44 calories per serving. You'll find this in the dietetic food section of your supermarket. Add salt—and why not a can of sliced mushrooms for taste, texture, richness? They're virtually a *no*-calorie food.

The other Diet-Pack soups aren't importantly lower in calorie count, their chief *raison d'être* apparently being that they're salt-free and sugar-free. Add salt and Lawry's Seasoned Salt to the Dorset mushroom or tomato soup, and they're really excellent. You may want to add half a Sucaryl tablet, too. Heinz or Campbell's Cream of Mushroom contains 30 calories per ounce, versus 11 calories in the Dorset Diet-Pack, so it's worth keeping on hand at all times.

See your shopping list of low-calorie items on pages 128–33 for other low-calorie soup ideas, such as borsch, onion soup, turtle soup, frozen Won Ton, and so on.

Fish to serve often
>Oyster cocktail
Oysters on the half shell
Oysters Rockefeller
Shrimp cocktail
Barbecued shrimps on cocktail skewers
Shrimp in cucumber mayonnaise*
Flaming shrimp
Crab-meat ramekins
Crab-meat cocktails

---

*Naturally, you use the de-calorized cream sauce for this.

Half a lobster in shell, cold or broiled
Clams on the half shell
Finnan haddie in ramekins*
Smoked salmon with fresh ground black pepper,
        lemon, capers
Smoked sturgeon, carp, or whitefish
Fillet of sole
Herring in sour cream
Bismarck herring
Fish balls on water cress
Sardine, lobster, or shrimp canapés
Steamed clams
Cold boiled salmon with green mayonnaise*
Mussels marinière
Cracked crab
Smoked shrimps, oysters or mussels
Scalloped tuna in ramekins*
Scalloped kebobs on cocktail skewers
Broiled rock lobster tails
Poached fillet (flounder, haddock, perch, etc.)
        with mushrooms or carrots and onions
Curried crab* in green pepper shells

A first course is a fine place to get more fish in
your family's diet, and thereby build up their metabolism and their intake of high-quality, low-cost protein.
If they're hearty eaters, and feel a little shortchanged
when the main course is fish, give it to them as an
extra course, that will fill but not fatten. Remember
that shellfish are packed with iodine which stimulates
your thyroid gland to speed up your metabolism, and
thereby burn up fat faster. Vitamins A, B, and D, and
fifteen other minerals beside iodine are packaged in
these fatless and flavorful tidbits, too.

Salad for a first course

Because you're going to use low-calorie dressings,
you'll have prepared them ahead of time, and have only
to pop them on your tray cart, ready to be added to
the salad at the table. Be sure to use the dark outer
leaves of the greens you buy; remember the greener

---

*Naturally, you use the de-calorized cream sauce for this.

they are, the richer they are in vitamin A, up to thirty times richer.

Lettuce with Thousand Island dressing
Greens with cottage cheese
Grapefruit, orange, and water cress
Tomato aspic with cottage cheese and/or bacon bits
Fresh spinach leaves and pineapple
Apple, celery, and shredded carrot
Thin sliced cucumbers, dusted with paprika in yogurt dressing
Chopped scallions and radishes, with greens, yogurt dressing
Lettuce, spinach, and endive, Roquefort dressing
Cucumber in aspic
Shredded, wilted lettuce with chopped crisp bacon
Caesar salad
Coleslaw with pineapple and English walnuts
Water cress, apricot, and cottage cheese
Fruits in aspic with sweetened mayonnaise
Waldorf salad

Buy a book of salads or send to *Good House-keeping* magazine for their excellent book of salads—and de-calorize.

Almost any salad will get way under the 100-calorie count per serving once you use the de-calorized dressing. Don't forget to use your pretty little molds, and serve individual aspics often. They're beautiful to look at and delicious to taste. Good source of protein, too, as well as vitamins.

Save dishwashing by stocking up on those individual salad-sized paper plates that look exactly like wooden plates.

Fruit first course favorites
Grapefruit, broiled with sherry or Marsala
Cantaloupe half, filled with cottage cheese
Honeydew with thin slices of prosciutto ham
Pear, or peach or apricot, filled with cottage cheese sprinkled with a few nuts
Fruit cups

Florida cocktail
Watermelon balls with chopped mint

Make a specialty of big fruit hors d'oeuvres plates from which people help themselves at table. Less work, more exciting to see and serve.

Make a watermelon "basket" by scooping out a pretty melon and keep it in your freezer all year, ready to take out and fill with various fruit mixes. After dinner, rinse it out and pop it back into the freezer again! Do the same with pineapples.

FAVORITE MAIN DISHES

Meats

There's just one reducer's rule in preparing meat dishes: *Get rid of the fat.**

The U.S. Department of Agriculture reports that studies just completed at the Indiana Experiment Station have established that the flavor of any meat is contained almost entirely *in the meat itself.* The bones rank a poor second; skin contributes even less than the bones. And the fat of any meat, including that of chicken, *contains virtually no flavor at all.*

How do you get rid of the fat? You can cut it off. You can also cook it off. You can leave out additional fat called for in preparing meat dishes. Or you can drastically reduce the amount in traditional recipes. To be specific:

1. Cut virtually *all* visible fat off meat before cooking. Yes, trim all but a film of it off *roasts,* too. The fat adds no flavor, remember. And if you weigh the amount of fat you've cut off, you can see that you've cut off plenty of calories at 250 calories per ounce!

---

*Look for low-fat cookery books in your library or bookstore for new ideas.

2. Use your broiler to brown meat: no fat required: does a good job too. If you pan-brown meat, instead of the two or three tablespoons of fat most recipes call for, merely brush the bottom of the heavy iron pan with oil. The purpose is to keep the meat from sticking to the bottom of the pan for that first quick minute of browning the surface. And a little does that job. The actual cooking of the meat over the flame should be done, without exception, over very low heat, if juiciness and delicious flavor are desired.

3. Fry in good oil, butter or margarine, but use it sparingly. *Fraction* the amount called for. You will find no flavor has been sacrificed by this. Measure what you use carefully and add in the calories; 36 per teaspoon.

4. Cook away the fat that's larded into pork and ham as much as possible. Fortunately these meats seem to get tastier and tastier the longer they are cooked . . . perhaps because the more fat cooked out of them, the more the good meat flavor predominates.

5. In utilizing leftover meats and fowl, use the low-calorie cream sauce on page 14. It's quick; it's easy, it's foolproof and delicious; and the calorie saving is 700 per cent over the traditional cream sauce.

6. Use the spray-on vegetable oil (PAM, for one); also Teflon-type pans for fat-free cooking.

Get rid of the fat and you can lose weight on any meat. Ham and pork? Certainly. Most diet books forbid them, I know, and prescribe steak and lamb chops as ℞-es for reducers. This is mysterious, since a pork chop contains 30% less calories than a lamb chop of the same weight.*

---

*Rib pork chop, 3 ounces, cooked without bone contains 284 calories; rib lamb chop, 3 ounces, cooked, without bone, contains 356 calories, according to the United States Department of Agriculture Handbook No. 8.

QUICK REFERENCE CHART of comparative calorie values of meat, fish, fowl

4 ounces without bone	approximate calorie count an average serving
lean fish shell fish canned sardines	80–100
chicken liver	125
tuna fish salmon	200
roast loin of pork veal cutlet, chops roast leg of veal lean tongue round steak, lean lean corned beef	200
pork chops ham spareribs roast beef duck Vienna sausages	250
roast turkey roast leg of lamb sirloin steak canned bulk sausages	300–400
lamb chops	480

Here is a rough calorie chart which you can use for quick reference as to the comparative calorie values of the various meats, fish, poultry.

You will see that some meats are lower in calorie count than others—chicken and lean fish lowest of all. You'll do well to serve these oftener than you used to. But the difference between one meat and another is not so great as to risk the setting of that fatal psychological trap; the tag on any meat of that alluring word: FORBIDDEN.

By cutting off all visible fat, and cooking off the built-in fat to some extent, you can easily reduce the calorie counts given here on fatty meats one-third.

Fat is not only flavorless, it's cheap. Butchers will give it away. Canners tend to load canned meat mixtures with it. So beware of canned chili con carne, stews, meat sauces, pork and beans, if you want to lose weight. They're calorie-loaded; and by making your own, using quick-easy recipes, you can eat twice or three times as much for no more calories.

More than 40 per cent of the average of America's calorie intake has been discovered to be *fat* calories. And more than half of these fat calories are hidden— in cooking grease, fats sopped up by meats, lard hidden in baking—fat that's slipped onto your waist and stomach while you're not looking, or tasting, or getting any pleasure out of it.

Even if you weren't trying to lose weight, your fat-calories should add up to less than 30 per cent of your daily intake, nutritionists agree. And a large part of that under-30 per cent should be liquid, *non*-hydrogenated fat. An excess of hydrogenated fat (fat in any *solid* form, including butter) seems definitely linked to arteriosclerosis—now the leading cause of death in men over 45.

It's horse-and-buggy thinking that *good* cooking equals *fat* cooking.

Chili Con Carne
Traditional recipe: 500 calories per serving
De-calorized recipe: 300 calories per serving

2 onions, diced
2 cloves garlic, minced
2 green peppers, diced
2 lbs. ground top-of-the-round, lean meat only
4 cups (No. 2½ can) tomatoes
4 cups canned kidney beans
⅔ tablespoon chili powder
⅔ teaspoon salt
2 teaspoons brown sugar

Sauté onions, garlic, and green peppers with meat in heavy iron pan. Add tomatoes, beans, and seasonings. Cover and simmer 20 minutes. Add a little water if mixture seems dry. Serves 8 to 10.

Pot Roast
Traditional recipe: 650 calories per serving
De-calorized recipe: 350 calories per serving

Brush bottom of heavy iron pan with a film of oil; wipe out any excess with a paper towel. Cut all fat off a 4-pound rump roast. Mix 2 tablespoons pastry flour with 1 teaspoon salt, black pepper, ¼ teaspoon ground ginger. Dust cut ends of roast with this; score meat by pushing a sharp-point knife through it at a right angle to the meat fibers, and at ½-inch intervals, in rows an inch apart.

Brown meat well on both sides; keep heat moderate, taking 15 to 20 minutes. Lift meat and set rack under it, then add ½ cup water, ½ cup tomato juice, 4 onions, each stuck with 2 cloves. Cover and put over extremely low heat. Simmer until almost tender, or about 3 to 4 hours. Remove meat, and whatever is left of onions and cloves. Add 1 cup of bouillon to liquid; season, if necessary; thicken with 1 tablespoon cornstarch which has been mixed with a little cold water. Serve this gravy with meat. If you wish vegetables with this—carrots, celery, onions, turnips, green pepper—peel and quarter them and put them in to cook with meat until tender, toward the end of the cooking period. Makes 8 to 10 servings.

Chow Mein

Traditional recipe: 350 calories per serving
De-calorized recipe: 200 calories per serving

    2 cups cooked, cleaned shrimps (pork, beef,
        ham, lobster, tuna, or chicken may be
        substituted)
    ½ cup scallions or onions, chopped
    1½ cups celery, sliced
    1 cup mushrooms, sliced
    1 teaspoon vegetable oil
    3 tablespoons soy sauce
    ½ teaspoon salt
    1 tablespoon cornstarch
    1 cup consommé or stock
    1 cup water chestnuts, sliced (optional)

Slice bunch of celery obliquely across into shreds. Slice shrimps through the back into halves. Put oil in skillet; stir shrimps into it for a minute. Add mushrooms, celery, scallions, soy sauce, and salt. Also water chestnuts, if used. Stir for 3 more minutes. Mix cornstarch, moistened with a little cold water, into the consommé; add to skillet and cook until the juice is translucent. Pour this on top of prepared Chinese or fried noodles, ¾ cup to a serving. Or if you wish to make noodles, boil 1 package fine noodles (8 to 9 ounces); drain and rinse. Heat 4 tablespoons vegetable oil in a big skillet. Divide the noodles into six portions. Roll up each portion like a shredded wheat biscuit. Fry until the outside is slightly browned but the inside is still soft. This can be done ahead of time and kept warm in the oven while preparing the chow mein. Serves 6.

Goulash
Traditional recipe: 450 calories per serving
De-calorized recipe: 250 calories per serving

     1 lb. round steak, or boneless beef chuck,
        cubed
     1 lb. lean veal, cubed
     1 lb. beef kidney, cubed
     1 teaspoon butter or margarine
     2 cups onions, thinly sliced
     ½ cup green pepper, diced
     2 teaspoons paprika
    1½ teaspoons salt
     ½ teaspoon pepper
     ½ teaspoon marjoram
    1½ cups tomatoes, canned
     2 cups potatoes, quartered
     1 cup carrots, diced

     Have meat cut in 1½-inch cubes. And cut
off fat left on cubes by butcher. In heavy iron pot
brown the meat quickly in the butter, with the
onions and peppers. Add all ingredients except
potatoes and carrots. Cover; simmer gently until
meat is tender, about an hour. Add a little water,
if necessary, and potatoes and carrots. Cook until
vegetables are tender. Serve with little dollops of
sour cream and parsley for garnish. Serves 8.

Beef Stroganoff
Traditional recipe: 450 calories per serving
De-calorized recipe: 325 calories per serving

     Buy 1½ pounds of lean round steak cut
½ inch thick; pound well, and cut with scissors
into strips ½ inch wide. Dredge by shaking in
paper sack containing 2 tablespoons seasoned
flour, ½ teaspoon paprika. In 1 tablespoon of
smoking hot vegetable oil, sear quickly. Add ½
cup tomato juice and sauté over low heat with
¾ cup of finely chopped onions, and 1 can of
sliced mushrooms. When meat is tender, add 1 cup
of yogurt or whipped cottage cheese, and serve as
soon as heated through. Serves 4.

Duck à L'orange
Traditional recipe: 325 calories per serving
De-calorized recipe: 150 calories per serving

1 Long Island duckling, 5–6 lbs.
2 teaspoons crystallized ginger, slivered
1 tablespoon orange rind, grated
1 cup orange juice
2 tablespoons Marsala
1 cup chicken consommé
2 tablespoons lemon juice
pinch of rosemary
salt, and dash of cayenne

Ask your meat dealer to skin the duckling and prepare for broiling. If you do it yourself (and it's easy since there is a solid layer of fat between the skin and meat) here's how: With a sharp knife, cut off wing tips; cut the skin from neck to vent, then along backbone. Loosen skin by running underneath close to flesh of duck. Peel skin back as it is loosened, cutting skin where necessary but leaving flesh intact. Now cut your skinned, de-fatted duckling in quarters. Cut wings from breast quarters so pieces will be of similar thickness. Remove duck to 9-inch casserole. (Combine ingredients given above for sauce and cover duck with this sauce.) Cover tightly. Bake in moderate oven (350° F.) 1¼ hours. Garnish with thin orange wedges and slivered toasted almonds. Serves 6.

Veal Scallopini
Traditional recipe: 325 calories per serving
De-calorized recipe: 210 calories per serving

    1 lb. thin veal cutlets
    1 teaspoon butter or olive oil
    3 tablespoons Marsala or sweet sherry or
        dry vermouth
    1 clove garlic, minced
    1 small can sliced mushrooms
    1 teaspoon meat concentrate
    1 teaspoon chili sauce
    1 cup bouillon
    salt, freshly ground black pepper, bay leaf

Have veal pounded into very thin slices. Brown meat in the butter or olive oil in heavy iron skillet, quickly. Add Marsala, then other ingredients, which have blended, and the bay leaf. Cover; simmer over low flame until the meat is tender. Serve very hot garnished with thin lemon slices, which have been dusted with chopped parsley. Serves 4.

Corned Beef and Cabbage
Traditional recipe: 700 calories per serving
De-calorized recipe: 375 calories per serving

    2 lbs. corned beef   1 green pepper
    4 cups boiling water   2 cloves
    1 head cabbage   1 bay leaf
    2 onions   pepper

Cut onions into rings, also cleaned green pepper. After removing all fat, cover meat with water and add onion, green pepper, cloves, bay leaves, and salt and pepper to taste. Simmer over very low heat until meat is tender (about 3 hours). Add cabbage, cut into chunks. Cook another 15 minutes. Serve meat surrounded by cabbage; garnish with parsley. Makes 4 servings.

Veal Stew
Traditional recipe: 550 calories per serving
De-calorized recipe: 200 calories per serving

    2 lbs. veal shoulder
    4 cups boiling water
    1 bay leaf
1½ teaspoons salt
    5 or 6 peppercorns
⅛ teaspoon thyme
    2 onions, sliced
    3 carrots, sliced or diced
    1 cup celery, thinly sliced
    1 green pepper, sliced
    2 sprigs parsley

Use veal breast or shoulder. Have the meat cut in 3-inch pieces. Cut off all possible fat. Put meat in heavy iron pot and pour boiling water over it. Add bay leaf and seasonings. Cover and simmer over low heat for 1½ hours. Add vegetables and continue cooking until vegetables are crisp-tender. Remove meat and vegetables to hot platter. Thicken gravy, if desired, with a little cornstarch mixed with cold water. Serves 4. DRESS-UP TOUCH: Soak wild rice overnight and add it along with a can of button mushrooms a few minutes before removing stew from heat. Garnish with dollops of fluffy sour cream. Only 30 calories in a tablespoon.

Roast Beef Hash
Traditional recipe: 500 calories per serving
De-calorized recipe: 300 calories per serving

Remove any fugitive bits of fat and gristle from cold roast beef or steak. Put meat through grinder, or chop it fine. To 1 cup or more of meat, add 2 cooked potatoes (chopped), ½ cup of chopped onion, ¼ teaspoon celery salt, a dash of poultry seasoning, ¾ cup bouillon, salt and pepper to taste. Mix well, and if you like, add 1 teaspoon of Worcestershire sauce. Brush an iron skillet with oil, and turn hash into it. Cook slowly over a low flame about 15 minutes until hash is browned on the bottom; then put under

a broiler to brown the top. This makes a fairly
wet hash; if you like a dry hash use less bouillon
and shape into patties, which can be turned with
a spatula to brown both sides. Chopped green
pepper and/or finely shredded carrot, and/or
chopped celery may be added to the mix before
cooking. Serves 4.

Fried Chicken, or Chicken in a Basket

115 calories for 4-ounce serving (without bone)
versus 235 for same portion fried traditional way

Cut 3-pound fryer into serving pieces, unless
you've bought "parts." Rub each piece of chicken
all over with the inside of a lemon that has been
cut into quarters, squeezing juice out as you rub.

Then salt each piece liberally with Lawry's
Seasoned Salt, or onion salt, lifting the skin and
salting well underneath it. Sprinkle with freshly
ground black pepper. Put the pieces in a covered
dish and let chicken marinate overnight in the
refrigerator.

When you're ready to cook it, put about 1
teaspoon of butter in a heavy skillet and brown
the pieces lightly on all sides, pressing the chicken
down, then moving it around so that it doesn't
stick. As pieces brown, lift them out into a broad
flat casserole. If the pieces aren't very well or
evenly browned, don't worry, this will be done
later.

Into the brown, crusty remainder that sticks
to the bottom of the skillet, pour about ½ cup of
boiling water and scrape residue until all is blended
and the pan bottom is clean. Taste this mixture,
adding a little salt, and perhaps ½ teaspoon of
sugar . . . until it's nicely seasoned. Pour over the
browned chicken in the casserole.

Cover the casserole with aluminum foil
tightly and put it in the oven, set at 350°. Let it
bake there for 40 minutes. Remove aluminum
foil and bake 10 to 15 minutes longer, or until
chicken is as deep a golden brown as you like.

This is the best "fried" chicken I ever ate . . .
moist and tender on the inside, brown and crusty on

the outside. I suspect the seasoned salt and marinating is responsible for the extra good flavor the chicken develops in the oven.

You'll find it just as delectable cold as hot . . . real chicken perfection cooked with this light, ungreasy hand.

Perfect Tuna Casserole
153 calories per serving versus 290 made traditionally

> In one-quart casserole combine 1 can Dorset Diet-Pack cream of mushroom soup with salt, ½ cup skimmed milk, a scant cup, drained, of flaked tuna (7-ounce can), 1 cup drained cooked green peas. Garnish top with corn flakes. Bake in moderate oven (375°) for 25 minutes. Serves 4.

Spaghetti, noodles, macaroni, rice and potatoes
Vital calorie statistics re: this family

Macaroni*	½ cup cooked	105 calories
Spaghetti	½ cup cooked	110 calories
Egg Noodles	½ cup cooked	53 calories
Potatoes, diced	½ cup cooked	52 calories
Rice, brown or white	½ cup cooked	102 calories

Easy to draw your own conclusions as to what is the best calorie buy among the pastas—obviously noodles, which happily can often double for macaroni and spaghettini. And if you want to go in for pasta in its fancier shapes—thimbles, shells, twists, pepper grains, starlets, threads—you'll find all those, too, among the noodles—at half the calories. That's because noodles absorb more water in cooking. Call it spaghettini or macaroni; why not?

Rice isn't so sinful, you see; the calories are likely to be more concentrated in the butter you wet it with. Use some of the fine de-calorized sauces in this book

---

*Buitoni and other firms use the word macaroni in the generic sense including all sizes and shapes of pasta—spaghettis, lasagna, shells, twists, etc., as well as the flat ribbons we usually identify as macaroni.

instead, and you can serve rice, as well as potatoes, spaghetti, macaroni, as often as your family wishes.

Make your sauces plentiful and do your skimping on the starchy base . . . this is rich man's eating and also thin man's eating! The reason the traditional recipes reverse the emphasis is because of the poverty of the people with whom they originated. Who can afford much meat in Italy and China and India? But here in America these savory dishes are kind to the budget even when you lay on the lean beef in triple or quadruple the pitifully small quantity called for in the Old-Country recipes.

The rule for de-calorizing all of these is: subtract fat; multiply the sauce; diminish the amount of the starchy base. And don't spare the garnishings.

"Macaroni" and Cheese
162 calories per cupful versus 464 calories in traditional recipe

    1 package noodles (8 ounces)
    2 cups cream sauce (page 14)
 ½ lb. sharp Cheddar cheese, grated
 ½ teaspoon onion, powder
    1 teaspoon prepared mustard
    1 teaspoon Worcestershire sauce (optional)

Cook noodles, drain and rinse. Combine hot cream sauce, grated cheese, onion powder, mustard, and Worcestershire sauce, reserving a third of the grated cheese for topping. Add noodles. Place in a lightly oiled casserole. Top with grated cheese remaining, and a dash of paprika. Bake in a moderate oven about 20 minutes, or until browned. Makes 9 servings.

"Spaghetti" with Meat Sauce
256 calories per serving versus 500 calories in traditional recipe

    2 cups tomato sauce (see page 100)
    1 8-ounce can tomato paste
    1 cup water
    1 clove, garlic, put through garlic press
    2 cups chopped onions
 1½ teaspoons salt
  ½ teaspoon basil
  ⅛ teaspoon thyme
    1 teaspoon orégano
    1 teaspoon sugar
    1 lb. lean beef, ground
    1 package egg noodles (8 oz.)
Parmesan cheese

Combine all ingredients except the beef and the noodles; stir well together. Cover and simmer while you brown the ground beef in a heavy skillet, turning it occasionally until it has all changed color.

Combine beef and tomato sauce and let them simmer together while you boil the noodles with salt, until it's almost (but not quite) soft— *al dente*, as the Italians say—with just enough firmness left so that your teeth can feel the texture.

Pour sauce over each serving of noodles and pass the grated Parmesan cheese with it . . . even at about 30 calories per teaspoonful. (The calorie count given above allows for 3 teaspoons per serving.) Serves 9.

VEGETABLES AND SALADS

What vegetables can your overweights eat? All of them! The cheerless little lists of "permissible" vegetables that are a standard feature of diet books are discouraging. Turnip greens, beet tops, dandelion greens, mustard greens, collards, kale. How many times can you serve these and get away with it?

The important thing is to get your overweights to

eat a lot of vegetables and salads. They are wonderful "filler-uppers," and good calorie buys—once the fattening butter, hollandaise, mayonnaise are de-calorized. It's not the calories in the vegetables but the calories in the butter you put on them that you have to out-maneuver. You'll find a number of ideas for low-calorie vegetable sauces on page 15.

Most overweights have a tendency to prefer the concentrated foods—starches, bread and butter, the pastas, fat meats, big solid desserts. If you can just increase their intake of vegetables and salads, you'll do a lot to lessen their intake of the more calorie-packed items.

Obviously you aren't going to get very far with mustard greens as your bait! And your overweights *won't* be forced—not for long, anyhow! So make a shrewd and careful study of the salads and vegetables they like best—and have them often! Go sleuthing for new ways to fix their old favorites. Be on the lookout for new and festive-looking vegetables to serve, alluring new ways to serve them, new dishes to serve them in.

Ask yourself: How many vegetables can be stuffed? What are they? (There are ten I know of. Can you add more?)

How many vegetable stuffings do you know? Make a list of them: cheese, corn, hash, chopped beef, ham, veal, lamb, etc.

How many big-scale vegetables have you served in the last few weeks? Asparagus, broccoli, perhaps cabbage, but what about leeks, artichokes, snow-peas, big mushrooms, those long Italian sweet peppers, Chinese bean sprouts, eggplant, celeriac, baked Hubbard squash?

How long since you've made a big beautiful vegetable aspic? Have you gotten into a rut, where vegetables and salads are concerned?

Give yourself a little shaking up; quite consciously decide to serve an old favorite a new way, or discover a new dish, at least twice a week.

Ask your children for ideas, take a trip through your supermarket, and through the foreign sections of town; cross-examine your pots and pans and molds to see if you're neglecting some of them.

Here are a few recipes:

Pseudo-Sweet Potato Fluff
80 calories in a serving
versus 300 in its sweet-potato twin

    4 lbs. Hubbard squash, cooked and mashed*, or
    2 packages frozen mashed squash
   15 Sucaryl tablets
   ¼ cup water
   ½ teaspoon maple flavoring
   ¼ cup dietetic orange marmalade
   ¼ cup brown sugar
    1 teaspoon cinnamon
    1 teaspoon salt
    6 pecan halves
    3 marshmallows

Bake and mash squash, or if using frozen squash, thaw it in top of double boiler.

Dissolve Sucaryl tablets in hot water. Combine with mashed squash and all except last two ingredients. Stir until well blended. Pour into lightly oiled casserole. Cut marshmallows in half and dot them on top with pecan halves. Bake in 350° oven for half hour. Serves 8.

This is a big success, sweet, fragrant, and festive as a birthday cake. Why call it squash, when most people would rather think they were eating yams or sweet potatoes? Texture is the same, tastes and looks much the same.

Next time you roast a turkey for Thanksgiving or Christmas or a company dinner, serve this alongside, with cranberry sauce, and perhaps green beans, cooked

---

*Cut squash in halves, lengthwise. Remove seeds and stringy portion. Place cut side down on a rack in a shallow baking pan. Bake in a hot oven (400°) until tender, about 30 minutes. Remove from oven, scoop out pulp, and mash until smooth.

with smoked salt pork and/or boiled onions garnished with black walnuts.

Cheese-Stuffed Peppers
109 calories each

>   5 medium green peppers
>   2 egg whites
>   ½ cup corn flakes
>   1 teaspoon onion juice
>   ¼ teaspoon paprika
> 1½ cups cottage cheese
>   1 cup basic tomato sauce (see page 100)

Cut tops off peppers, clean out their innards. Parboil them if you like (I don't). Whip egg whites to a white froth, but not until stiff. Roll corn flakes with rolling pin to crumbs. Combine onion juice, paprika, corn flakes, egg whites, and cottage cheese. Fill peppers with mixture and set them in a shallow baking dish into which you have already put the tomato sauce. Bake covered for 30 minutes in 350° oven. A few minutes before serving, top each pepper with a dab of wine-Cheddar cheese and put back into the oven until it melts. This is a real *bonne bouche*—fresh, delicate in both taste and texture. Pretty to look at, too.

Sweet Corn Pudding
a mere 94 calories per serving
(who says corn is so fattening?)

To 1 can of cream-style corn add ¼ cup evaporated skimmed milk, ¾ cup of water. Into a saucepan empty contents of one envelope of Tasti-Diet butterscotch pudding mix; stir until smooth. Gradually add the rest of the liquid, the corn, salt to taste, a dash of pepper.

Cook over medium heat, stirring constantly until the mixture comes to a boil and has thickened. Add more salt, if necessary. Pour into a lightly oiled casserole. Top with a sprinkle of toast crumbs and paprika. Keep in a warm oven until ready to serve. Serves 5. (Wonderful with ½ cup of dried chipped beef added while it is thickening; and only 33 calories more per serving.) Serve the plain corn pudding with cold sliced tongue and a green salad and you have the makings for a fine summer's night supper.

If you prefer a less sweet corn pudding, mix drained canned corn with low-calorie cream sauce (see page 14), and sprinkle brown sugar over the top. Bake in a casserole for 30 minutes in moderate oven.

Don't forget to try artichokes and/or hearts of palm with that heavenly low-calorie hollandaise on page 21. Make an opening course of it. Only 90 calories in a whole 15-ounce can of hearts of palm. Artichoke hearts come frozen now, too.

Don't forget that mushrooms are almost a no-calorie vegetable; luxurious, delicate, delicious. Stuff them, scallop them, cream them, devil them. Combine them with other vegetables and/or meat.

Two simple, but delightful, ways to serve mushrooms

1. Wash and slice fresh mushrooms, put them in a skillet with a clove of garlic and some salt, pepper, and Ac'cent. Cover and cook for a few minutes over low heat. The mushrooms cook in their own juice and are very tasty. Serve as is or—

2. When the mushrooms are cooked, add light sour cream—just enough to moisten mushrooms well. Thirty calories per tablespoon—only three calories more than in a tablespoon of yogurt or cottage cheese. Heat just until cream is warmed through, and serve. (Take out the garlic clove first, though!)

There are many intriguing ideas and recipes in the magazines for new vegetables dishes. And they're easy to revise, once you're on guard against the high-calorie ingredients, and know the basic sauces given here.

So take over! Start a collection. There are only a few meats, but there are literally dozens of vegetables you can corral for new cooking adventures, and pleasurable reducing.

The much-maligned potato

Again, it's not so much the potato, but the fat that's served with it, that does the figure-damage. A potato soaks up grease like a blotter. But contrive to serve potatoes that aren't carrying a great freight of fat. They should be on your menus often, if your family is fond of them. A baked potato carries fewer calories than a roll, and has a lot more nutrition to contribute.

Your de-calorizing techniques with potatoes are basically three:

1. Make a little potato look big. *Get out that potato ricer;* it fluffs an ounce of potato into three times its original bulk. Riced potatoes look "party-fied," too, have prestige value.
   Serve potato balls made with your biggest melon baller. *Use your electric mixer* or beater to whip air into boiled potatoes to which you've added hot skimmed milk, a bit of grated onion, salt and pepper. Aerated potatoes swell noticeably in bulk.
   Use your pastry tube to make potato borders out of the aerated potatoes.

2. When you use butter, put it *all* where it shows. Put a thin square of butter on top. For the heavy moistening work, have a pitcher of fatless meat juice to pass quickly. Men love good meat juices. And they needn't contain much more fat than water. Don't forget that good low-calorie Franco-American Beef Gravy, as an alternate.

3. Serve potatoes in a prefabricated moisture which need contain no butter at all. Using the de-calorized cream sauce on page 14, you can serve, for example, these three big favorites: creamed potatoes; au gratin potatoes; scalloped potatoes. Using Low-May (mayonnaise), well-seasoned according to the family's taste, have potato salad as often as you like.

SAUCES AND SALAD DRESSINGS

Made the traditional way, they're *murder*. It's appalling to consider how many hidden calories they conceal. When your 30 calories worth of cauliflower wears the traditional cheese sauce it contains 180 calories, suddenly. With hollandaise, it jumps from 30 to 230. Even a thin pink blanket of innocent-looking tomato sauce made the traditional way adds over 100 calories to whatever it surrounds. A sundae can contain two or three times as many calories as ice cream alone. As for mayonnaise, it's an open secret that it's as fattening as butter.

Dressings and sauces can, on occasion, be very important to our enjoyment of salads and vegetables. Yet they're so almost invisible, that even people who eat lightly to keep their weight down, end by loading in thousands of calories worth of these bodiless moistenings every month.

Needlessly! Because it's so easy to *keep* flavor and *lose* calories in these sauces and salad dressings. You can buy most of them ready-made. Use them as is, or add your own seasonings. If the flavor and texture are the same, who's so anxious to keep the calories?

Half the battle, in fool-the-scale cookery, is mastering the secrets of de-calorizing sauces and salad dressings. Nothing, but nothing, is more important. *De-calorized sauces are terrific "save-sies" for the twentieth-century cook.*

You, and yours, certainly don't want a sauce on everything. Perhaps most of the time you prefer your dishes unsauced, except with their own good juices.

But—what about that hollandaise on spring's first asparagus? The creamy-bite-y horseradish sauce on boiled beef? The tartar sauce with scallops or fillet of sole? Chocolate sauce on ice cream for chocolate lovers? Most people feel they add a lot.

And in making leftover roasts and vegetables a treat instead of a dismal duty, don't you agree that a good cream sauce, and its various flavorful cousins, are pretty basic?

Here are the three big reasons for learning to de-
calorize your sauces and salad dressings—but *quick*.

1. *Your cooking won't seem like "diet cooking."*
Try to put your family (or yourself) on a one hundred per cent sauceless diet, and sooner or later they're
likely to rebel, because they're feeling shortchanged
on trimmings and eating fun. The frequent sight and
taste of their favorite sauces prevents this.

2. *Butter sauce is the downfall* of many a weight-
watcher. It *seems* such a nothing. De-calorized sauces
and dressings at 10 to 20 calories per tablespoon
can save thousands of butter and salad-oil calories—
enough to mean easily 5 to 10 pounds in, say, six
months. Keep track one day and figure it out for
yourself. You have to keep count to *believe* how many
calories sneak up on you in melted butter.

3. *Your cooking repertoire is unlimited.* Without
benefit of sauces and salad dressings your cooking may
be good, but it's going to be monotonous. Learn to de-
calorize them, and those holiday feasts, parties, and
company dinners (they add up in a year!) won't mean
that everybody's calorie intake has to go sky-high
again.

Your sauces are as personal as your wardrobe—
don't give them up! Just modernize them.

For any kind of meat, fish, poultry, hot or cold;
for any kind of vegetable, any kind of salad, you have
only to get acquainted with de-calorizing seven simple
sauce bases.

You can make seven *times* seven sauces from
these bases; as easy as falling off a log. They're the
bases of substantially all sauces. Different spicings in
tropical dishes than in Scandinavian, but the seven
starting points are pretty much the same. Here they
are:

1. cream sauce base (hot)
2. tomato sauce base
3. chilled cream dressing
4. mayonnaise base
5. hollandaise base

6. French dressing base
7. brown sauce or gravy base

Let's take them one at a time and see what calorie cuts can be made without changing their character.

1. Cream sauce base

39 calories—or 215 calories in your serving?

See page 14, for the quick, easy, low-calories recipe for cream sauce and *umpteen* variations thereof; for cheering and cozying up meats, fish, vegetables, chicken; for adding zest to leftovers; for simplifying soufflés, curries, and other culinary complexities.

If you like a thick blanket of savory cheese sauce over your cauliflower, for instance, read how you can have it for 50 calories, instead of 180 (page 15).

Don't forget to keep Dorset Diet-Pack Cream of Mushroom Soup on hand when you need a mushroom-flavored cream sauce and don't have even five minutes to make one in. It's salt-free, so you'll need to add extra salt. But flavored up a bit with Lawry's Seasoned Salt and sherry, it's very acceptable. Not as good as the traditional cream of mushroom soup you may have been using to pinch-hit for cream sauce; but Dorset's only contains 11 calories per ounce versus 30 calories per ounce of the regular cream of mushroom soup. So keep it handily at the front of your soup shelf; and if you have any of the regular caloric variety on hand, return it to the grocer or give it away; *get it out of the house.*

2. Tomato sauce base

46 to 90 calories per cup—or 314 calories when made traditionally?

Traditional tomato sauce recipes demonstrate nicely the needlessness of the fat that's packed into so many old-time recipes. Why should a tomato sauce be greasy? Its purpose in a recipe is to season and moisten. The 4 to 6 tablespoons of oil that the old-fashioned recipes call for add nothing to the light brightness of its flavor. The pungent flavor of olive oil will not be missed, because the garlic, oregano, and onion used are so much more pungent.

For one low-calorie tomato sauce, follow the traditional recipe in your cookbooks; substitute Sucaryl for sugar and leave out the fat (46 to 50 calories per cup).

Wonderfully worksaving and almost as low-calorie is Hunt's Tomato Sauce, which contains no high-calorie ingredients except a mite of sugar (or rather dextrose which amounts to the same thing). One 8-ounce can contains 90 calories—a very good calorie buy—and a thick, flavorful, even-textured sauce that can be used as is, if you're partial to bland food. Or seasoned and varied from now till Kingdom Come.

Basic Quick Tomato Sauce
(46 calories per cup)

    1 bouillon cube
1½ cups water
    4 Sucaryl tablets
½ cup onion, chopped
    1 clove garlic, put through garlic press
        (optional)
small piece bay leaf
    2 8-ounce cans Hunt's Tomato Sauce
½ teaspoon celery salt

Dissolve bouillon cube in water with Sucaryl tablets in a skillet. Add onion, garlic, bay leaf, and cook 2 minutes. Add tomato sauce and celery salt, cook. Makes almost 3 cupfuls of sauce.

Creole Sauce (or Spanish Sauce)
(100 calories per cup)

To quick basic tomato sauce, add ½ cup green peppers, chopped, 1 teaspoon chili powder, ⅛ teaspoon ground cloves, ½ cup stuffed olives (optional). Add these ingredients with onions and garlic to the bouillon mixture you start with.

Use this sauce to bake fish fillets; to make

Shrimps Creole (simply warm the cooked, de-veined shrimps in it); in omelets; with green beans, eggplant, lima beans, spinach; as a sauce on stuffed green peppers, stuffed onions, stuffed summer squash, etc. Bake pork chops in it; use it as a sauce over meat loaf, on Swiss steak, for goulash. It's as widely useful, almost, as cream sauce.

Clam-Tomato Sauce
(130 calories per cup)

Add one 7-ounce can of minced clams, and clam liquor to basic tomato sauce recipe given above. Serve with spaghetti.

3. Chilled cream dressing
28 calories in your serving—or 120?

Cream, or thinned, whipped cream cheese is the traditional base; combined with lemon or vinegar and seasonings. Unfortunately these bodiless cream "drippings" add almost as many calories as mayonnaise to your serving of the salad, fish, or aspic.

This *needn't* be so. Use fluffy white yogurt, without changing either flavor or texture, you cut the calories about 75 per cent. Dannon, bless them, have de-calorized their yogurt; delicious, too!

Basic de-calorized cream dressing
28 calories per serving

  1 cup yogurt, sour cream, or evaporated
      skimmed milk (for a whipped cream
      texture, use whipped cottage cheese)
  3 tablespoons lemon juice
  ½ teaspoon salt
  1 teaspoon Lawry's Seasoned Salt
  ½ teaspoon garlic salt

Stir well together; add flavor variations to suit your taste buds and the dish you're "dressing" with this snowy, fresh-tasting cream.

A few "for instances":

With cold salmon: add ½ cup of the pale yellow prepared mustard. This makes a mustard "mayonnaise" of a spirited lightness that beats the heavy conventional mayonnaise all hollow.

With fish aspics: add 1 teaspoon fresh chopped dill, and ½ cup of cucumber shavings. A fresh delicacy, and a textural interest, this has; somehow a soul mate for almost any fish. Garnish with capers.

As a cocktail sauce for chunks of cold lobster, crab, or shrimp: add ½ cup of chili sauce; 1 tablespoon horseradish; ½ teaspoon dry mustard; tabasco sauce.

With coleslaw, fruit salads, or aspics: substitute ½ cup of grapefruit or pineapple juice for the lemon juice; sweeten with 1 teaspoon honey.

With boiled beef: use only 1 tablespoon lemon juice, in basic recipe; add 2 tablespoons fresh horseradish.

On green salads: use as is, or plus garlic croutons, for texture interest; or crumbled crisp bacon; or torn-up anchovies. Or you can make it *Russian* dressing in two shakes by adding chili sauce.

This doesn't begin to exhaust the possibilities of this luscious low-calorie, high-protein sauce. Add celery seed or caraway seeds, India relish, Worcestershire sauce, chopped parsley, chopped stuffed olives, chopped radishes, and curry powder; not to mention raisins, nuts, chopped apples, chopped kumquats in the sweet and sour versions.

4. Mayonnaise or salad dressing base
      5 calories per tablespoon—or 92?

At the supermarket you have the choice of buying

(a) traditional mayonnaise, at 92 calories per tablespoon
(b) salad dressing at 58 calories per tablespoon
(c) the low-calorie mayonnaise in the dietetic food section, which contains about 5 calories per tablespoon!

Sauce maison, sans avoirdupois: (This is the stand-by and creation of my friend Jane Levy, who is one of the plain-and-fanciest good cooks I know.) Low-May base, to which she adds, to taste: chili sauce, chopped parsley, capers, India relish, Ac'cent, pepper, Beau Monde seasoning, horseradish, onion powder, celery seed, English mustard, garlic salt, tabasco, Worcestershire—and salt to taste.

Basic Phantom Mayonnaise: 16 calories per tablespoon. Follow recipe for hollandaise on page 21 using 2 tablespoons lemon juice, 4 tablespoons water, ½ teaspoon dry mustard, ¼ teaspoon onion powder. Good—and good for you. Not as smooth as mayonnaise, but in a salad, who'd know? *And digest this:* traditional mayonnaise contains 440 grams of fat, 5.6 grams of protein: this, only 2 grams of fat, 50 of protein!

Quick barbecue sauce: Mix together

⅔ cup tomato ketchup
½ cup Phantom mayonnaise
1 tablespoon mustard-with-horseradish sauce

Spread on split frankfurters, hamburgers, other meat or chicken before broiling. Spoon excess sauce over meat while cooking.

Use it hot, on vegetables, instead of butter sauce. Vary with a bit of added curry powder, or prepared mustard, or Worcestershire sauce. Use it on boiled, poached or baked fish, plus chopped fresh dill, and/or chopped cucumbers. Use it on cold meats and meat salads, plus prepared mustard.

Russian dressing: Put cold mayonnaise in your electric beater with ⅓ cup chili sauce, 2 tablespoons chopped sweet pickle, to 1 cup mayonnaise.

Whipped Cream Dressing: In a small bowl put ¼ cup water, 2 tablespoons lemon juice, 1 tablespoon dry skimmed milk. Beat in electric beater until stiff. Fold into 1 cup mayonnaise.

Orange Whipped Cream Dressing: Fold 2 teaspoons grated orange rind and 2 tablespoons orange juice into whipped cream dressing.

5. Hollandaise base
351 calories per cup—or 1250 calories?

If you like hollandaise the way I do, you don't even want to hear how many calories there are in a tablespoonful. Because what good is a mingy table-spoonful? Even ¼ cupful makes a stingy little blob over a serving of broccoli or cauliflower or asparagus. Half a cup isn't a bit too much—it goes down in a few ecstatic moments. Calorie cost: 625 calories. Let's face it, a quarter of all the calories we "burn" in a day!

That's why I figure the recipe on page 21 is a master recipe and worth the price of the book several times over. Because this de-calorized hollandaise is of a beautiful goldenness; of a cloudlike lightness; with a flavor that really sings a high note.

And the oftener you serve your vegetables well-lathered with this lip-smacking sauce, the better! There isn't a calorie of fat in a carload of it. There are calories, but they are 99.44 per cent pure protein.

6. French dressing base
1 calorie per tablespoon—or 59 calories?

Fifty-nine calories in one tablespoon of most traditional French dressings. But you can buy a twentieth-century French dressing in your dietetic food section that's *one* calorie per tablespoon. It's called Frenchette dressing. Try it on hot green beans as well as salad; also on spinach or any other greens. Add lemon or salt if you find it too sweet.

This is just one of the low-calorie French dressings, even more numerous than the dietetic mayonnaises. Worth tinkering with—and they *need* plenty!

Or you can make your own French dressing with unhydrogenated oil—a good way to get your 1 to 2 tablespoonfuls. Look for an olive-y tasting oil called Lettuce Leaf Oil.

7. Brown sauce or gravy base

Only 4 calories per tablespoon, versus 40 to 90 calories for traditionally made beef gravy or brown sauce.

(They're basically the same; browned fat and flour, liquid and seasonings.)

Gravy is a bit of extra bother, and so fattening that calorie-conscious America is making less and less of it. How fattening it is, largely depends, of course on how much fat goes into it.

But gravy is a cozy thing, with potatoes, on flank steak (a wonderful calorie buy and an elegant meat) —in using beef leftovers.

Men love it. And now there's no reason on earth why it shouldn't appear on your table, because the Campbell Soup Company, blessed be their name, have put out a twentieth-century beef gravy in a can. The brand name is Franco-American.

All you do is heat and eat. The flavor is nice, the price is right.

Just as you get it from the can, a tablespoon contains 8 calories—little enough. But I like to spike the flavor up a bit, adding one-half teaspoon of Worcestershire sauce to the can and quite a bit of garlic salt. Then I found that if I diluted it with an equal amount of water and added some Gravy Master and Maggi Seasoning, I had just as beefy a gravy; thinner, but still not too thin; and half the calories.

We like a thin gravy, so this suited me and mine. It may not suit you and yours; but at 4 calories or 8 calories in a tablespoon, this is still a wonderful addition to your supply shelf of low-calorie staples; a great substitute for butter on potatoes.

You'll think of dozens of ways this good beef gravy can save you work and weight-gaining; as a sauce for kidneys, liver—those good oomph-loaded organ meats—with a little red wine added; in stews and meat pies; on noodles; with meat balls; as moistening for roast-beef hash; as a dressing for boiled onions; as a topping on meat-stuffed vegetables. Keep a can of it right at the front of your supply cupboard and remember about it. It's a new convenience, and it's easy to forget to use these new ways.

One more sauce

The most popular fruit-flavor sauce is fortunately one that de-calorizes sensationally—cranberry sauce. Traditional recipe, 139 calories to ¼ cupful; de-calorized version, 24 calories per ¼ cupful.

Cranberry sauce (traditional recipe)

1 lb. cranberries, raw	218 calories
2 oranges, small	100 calories
2 cups sugar	1,748 calories
	2,066 calories

de-calorized recipe

1 lb. cranberries, raw	218 calories
2 oranges, small	100 calories
40 tablets Sucaryl	00 calories
1 tablespoon sugar	48 calories
	366 calories

Why not all Sucaryl? I don't know. But it *tasted* better when I used exactly 1 tablespoon of sugar— and I've tried it with half a dozen different amounts of sugar . . . as well, of course, as without any. As a matter of fact, this makes a rather sweet cranberry sauce; you might start with 30 Sucaryl tablets if you like a tart sauce. You can always add more.

Procedure: Put raw cranberries and fresh oranges, skin and all, through a food grinder. Dissolve Sucaryl tablets in ½ cup hot water. Combine all ingredients and marinate at least 3 hours in refrigerator. Refrigerated, this sauce keeps a week or more.

Suggestion: Keep cranberry sauce in your refrigerator and serve it *often*, with meat as well as turkey and chicken. It's so wonderfully low-calorie, and yet satisfies that sweet tooth; makes a tart-sweet, fresh-tasting contrast to cold lamb, for instance, or with curries (on the chutney principle) as well as with chicken and turkey.

Take a flyer in flavors

Since it's in sauces that flavors get star-billing, find yourself some new ones! There are more flavors to be had than your supermarket shelf tells you. And why shouldn't twentieth-century kitchen cooks have the fun and advantages of playing with them, as well as industrial chefs and big bakeries? You *need* flavors, you *don't* need calories.

Look in your classified directory under FLAVORING EXTRACTS. Chances are you'll find a nice little clutch of names and addresses, some perhaps, forbiddingly called laboratories or chemical companies . . . but *investigate!*

In New York, a great many of these flavoring extract companies are tiny shops, run by a nice Italian family, who clearly are descendants of the old-time alchemists. You'll see rows and rows of small bottles, and are given a catalogue listing a couple of hundred flavors. The list that follows is from the Insuperable Extracts Company, 409 East 116 Street, a tiny place. This is only a third of the flavors they carry.

For very little money I also carried home about twenty little bottles of unheard-of new flavors to try. If Insuperable was out of a flavor I asked for, some member of the family nipped into a back room, quickly put it together, and Mama wrapped it up for me.

Have you tried these bottled flavorings? Apple, Apricot, Avocado, Banana, Bay Leaves, Blackberry, Bourbon, Burnt Almond, Butter, Butterscotch, Caraway, Cardamom, Carnation, Celery, Cantaloupe, Carrot, Wild Cherry, Cheese, Chocolate, Cinnamon, Citron, Clove, Coconut, Cola, Coriander, Cranberry,

Crême de Cacao, Crême de Menthe, Currant, Curry,
Date, Dill, Elder Flowers, Fennel, Fig, Garlic, Gin,
Ginger, Gooseberry, Grape, Grapefruit, Guava, Ha-
zelnut, Honey, Horehound, Jasmine, Licorice, Loganberry, Mace, Maple Walnut, Maywine, Nutmeg, Orange blossom, Paprika, Peach, Pear, Pecan, Papaya,
Passion Fruit, Pepper, Plum, Port wine, Quince, Raspberry, Root beer, Rum & Butter, Rum & Maple, Sassa-
fras, Sweet Basil, Tutti Frutti, Violet, Vodka.

Some of these flavors are fantastic! When I open
that tiny bottle of raspberry, for example, my whole
kitchen is perfumed with the odor of fresh raspberries.
When I open the cassis extract bottle, the kitchen smells
of currant jelly. The nut flavors are very successful,
too. In fact, I never got so much cooking pleasure and
adventure out of so little money in my life.

DESSERT FAVORITES

If you've fed your overweights properly, by dessert time their interest in food should spring more from
a desire for pure pleasure than from hunger pangs. But
that's no reason for cheating them out of their sweets.
On the contrary, it's the best of reasons for making
sure they get them because, of all foods and drinks,
sweets are the most heavily charged with emotional
dynamite—at least for most of America. From childhood we carry over a reflex association of sweets with
reward for good behavior, with Mother's approval, with
our birthday parties, holiday feasts, and other especially happy, emotional times.

This is the bigger half of the reason why sweets are
so often the downfall of would-be reducers. The rest
of the reason why sweets so often lick us is that
they're such terrific concentrations of calories: 300 to
600 calories in most of the desserts America loves
best—pie, ice-cream sundaes, chocolate layer cakes,
strawberry shortcake.

But just as this is an age of miracle fabrics and
wonder drugs, it's an age of phantom foods, and high

time, too, considering the rate at which we're losing the male population over forty!

Saccharin and Sucaryl rank first among the modern man-made miracles in the pseudo-food department —nary a calorie in a carload—as opposed to the 768 calories *one cup* of sugar contains.

De-calorized desserts will not do the rest of the family any injustice. Your de-calorized whips, for instance, give them a lot more of what they need even more than calories—far more vital body nutrients. Whipped evaporated skimmed milk, for example, contains six times as much protein and calcium as whipped cream; whipped cottage cheese, eight times as much protein as whipped cream.

And learning to de-calorize desserts so that you can serve big beautiful helpings is important. Robbed, or skimped, when it comes to dessert, for lack of a feeling of satiation, you are likely to see your overweight dipping absentmindedly into a box of chocolates that has appeared mysteriously in the house from nowhere.

Popular delusions about ice cream—America's first love:

1. That water ice has fewer calories than ice cream.

   Fact: ½ cup of orange water ice contains 177 calories, ½ cup of vanilla ice cream, 147 calories.

   Conclusion: Not always. Though orange ice contains more calories than most water ices.

2. That vanilla ice cream has the fewest calories among ice creams.

   Fact: Coffee ice cream has almost 100 calories less per pint than vanilla.

Conclusion: Nice if you like coffee ice cream.

3. That chocolate is the most fattening of the ice
     creams.

Fact: ½ cup of chocolate ice cream contains 358
        calories.
        ½ cup of peach ice cream contains 420 cal-
        ories.

4. That there isn't enough difference in the calorie
     count of different ice creams to matter
     much.

Fact: Frozen Nesselrode pudding contains about
       600 calories per serving!

Conclusion: Your best calorie buys among the
             commercial ice creams are:

      raspberry ice, at 117 calories per half cup
      most commercial sherbets, 118 calories per
            half cup
      coffee ice cream, 125 calories per half cup
      vanilla ice cream, 147 calories per half cup

If you eat a lot of ice cream, the flavor you pick
can add up to a big calorie difference over a long, hot
summer.

By the time you read this, an enlightened dairy
industry may have come out with an honest-to-gosh
low-calorie ice cream. But don't believe it unless the
ads give you the actual calorie count; and no such
specious comparisons as "less than in a glass of prune
juice," either. I have seen "low-calorie" ice cream in
the supermarket, but when I wrote the makers for the
calorie count, it turns out to contain 523 calories per
pint of vanilla ice cream. Since regular ice cream contains about 588 calories per pint of vanilla, I don't
consider this amounts to enough of a saving per serving
to be worth mentioning.

If you're all ice cream lovers, write to the maker for calorie counts.

Even at 588 calories to the pint, ice cream is much too good to give up. You'll read here how to make de-calorized ice cream that contains only 40 to 50 calories per ½ cup serving, instead of the 147 calories in commercial vanilla flavor. But that de-calorized product may not always be available.

Problem: how can you make *less* ice cream seem like *more* ice cream?

Lightweight Approach

1. Use a big melon-baller and serve ice cream in a pretty cluster of globes, like giant grapes. This way a half cup looks like a fairly big serving.

Get a small-sized ice-cream scoop. The plastic ones with efficient pop-it-out squeeze handles, hold only 2 tablespoons (⅛ cup). Even the regulation size metal ice-cream scoop holds only ⅓ of a cup of ice cream. But this is when you level the ice cream off across the flat of the scoop; so that while it looks like a baseball of ice cream, it sits on a flat bottom. The important thing is to fill your scoop with water and find out *exactly* how much it does hold; with a half cup of vanilla "costing" about 150 calories, you need to establish clearly in your mind, once and for all, just how much you're serving with each scoop.

2. Serve something beneath the ice cream; fruit, meringue, a thin slice of angel cake and more of the same on top of it. Make as big-looking a structure as possible.

3. Make a specialty of stylish ice-cream desserts. The more uptown it looks, the bigger it tastes.

De-Calorized Ice Cream, 40 to 50 calories per half cup versus 147 calories per half cup for store-bought vanilla ice cream.

Step one: Dissolve 6 Sucaryl tablets in 2 table-spoons boiling water. Dissolve 1 en-velope sugar-free D-Zerta Gelatin (any flavor) in the same boiling water. Let cool.

Step two: Sprinkle a little salt on two egg whites which are room temperature. Beat until frothy; add ¼ teaspoon vinegar and beat until stiff. Add 2 tablespoons sugar and beat a few minutes longer.

Step three: Whip chilled evaporated skimmed milk until it begins to stiffen; then add 4 tablespoons lemon juice, and 1 tablespoon sugar and beat until stiff. (Use 6 ounce can of milk.)

Step four: Fold egg whites and Jell-o mixture into milk. Stir in 1 teaspoon vanilla. Pour into ice cube tray and put back in freezing compartment to firm.

Variations: Instead of vanilla, add 1 teaspoon angostura bitters just before freezing. Or maple flavoring. Or 1 tablespoon maraschino cherry juice and ¼ cup chopped maraschino cherries. Or 1 tablespoon very strong instant coffee, Sucaryl sweetened, if you like. Or 1 medium, *very* ripe banana, mashed. Or ¼ cup crushed peanut brittle. Or ¼ cup shredded coconut. Or marble with Choc-Low by stirring 2 table-spoons warmed Choc-Low through mixture when it is half-frozen, using a knife for stirring. Or stir in ¼ cup of any concentrated sugarless fruit syrup "matching" fresh fruit.

This has a slightly different taste and texture than store-bought ice cream, as any homemade ice cream has; lighter, less fatty, but definitely creamy neverthe-less. Because of the enormous calorie saving, it's very much worth trying. If you have a freezer, you can make it up in quantity in different flavors that the family favor, and have it always on hand for a wholesome, high-protein, low-calorie between-meals and bedtime snack.

It's especially worth while when there are children whose weight must be watched, as this ice cream can be used in floats, milk shakes, frosted coffees, ice-cream cones, etc. This recipe makes between 5 and 6 cups of ice cream—as much as 1½ quarts—depending on the size of the egg whites and the volume you get in beating both egg whites and milk.

As you see, some of the variations suggested will add calories, but the number per serving is not likely to amount to more than 10, so the sky's the limit on variations!

And don't forget the garnishings: more fresh fruit on top, crushed nuts, coconut, whipped "cream," a cherry, or chocolate sprinkles—whatever your family considers most luxurious.

Plum Ring
99 calories per serving.

1 can Diet-Sweet Purple Plums
1 envelope Knox's Gelatin
½ cup cold water
1 teaspoon lemon juice
2 tablespoons black raspberry sugarless beverage mix
½ teaspoon cassis flavoring
¾ cup evaporated skimmed milk

Soften gelatin in cold water. Combine with rest of ingredients. Pour into ring mold. Put in refrigerator to set. Chill skimmed milk until almost frozen, and then whip it until stiff. Sweeten with Sucaryl. Unmold ring and fill center with whipped milk. Dust with grated orange peel before serving. Serves 6.

Green Grape Compote
132 calories per serving.

> For each person . . .
> 30 little green grapes
> 1 tablespoon honey
> 1 tablespoon lemon juice

Let marinate overnight; just before serving, top with 1 tablespoon sour cream.

Zabaione or Zabaglione
97 calories per serving.

> For each person . . .
> 1 egg yolk
> 1 teaspoon sugar
> half the eggshell filled with Marsala wine

Put in top of double boiler; stir well. Beat over boiling water until fluffy and thick. Take out of boiling water, continue stirring with a spoon. Serve hot or chilled with a dash of nutmeg.

Banana Flambé Kirsch
123 calories per serving.

> For each person . . .
> 1 small banana
> ½ teaspoon sweet butter
> ½ teaspoon brown sugar
> 1 tablespoon kirsch, gin, or vodka

Butter a copper pan; split peeled banana lengthwise and sprinkle with sugar. Cover and simmer over a very low fire for 15 minutes. Just before serving throw kirsch over banana; set it on fire.

15-minute De-calorized Cheesecake
100 calories per serving
versus 400 calories per serving in traditional recipe.

Start by putting one 6-ounce can of evaporated skimmed milk in the freezing compartment to chill.

Step one: put 2 envelopes of Knox's unflavored gelatin in ¼ cup cold water.

Step two: fill another cup with water. In a small saucepan empty contents of one en-

velope D-Zerta vanilla pudding. Add
1 tablespoon water from the cup and
mix well. Add remainder of the cup
of water. Cook over medium heat,
stirring constantly until it comes to a
boil. Add 42 Sucaryl tablets. Take
off fire, and add softened gelatin. Stir
until well blended. Let cool.

Step three: into electric blender put 2½ cups
cottage cheese, and 1 teaspoon grated
lemon rind, 2 tablespoons lemon juice,
and cooled custard mixture. Blend
until smooth, about 1 minute.

Step four: beat whites of two eggs until stiff.

Step five: beat chilled evaporated milk with 2
tablespoons lemon juice until stiff.
Add 1 teaspoon vanilla, ½ teaspoon
almond extract.

Step six: fold egg whites and whipped milk
into custard cheese mixture and turn
into 8-inch spring-form pan. Sprinkle
top with mixture of crumbs of graham
crackers which have been mixed with
½ teaspoon cinnamon, 1 teaspoon
sugar, a good dash of nutmeg, and
then with 1 teaspoon melted butter.
Chill until firm (at least 4 hours).

This wonderfully simplified recipe yields 9 servings. Nine hundred calories in the whole cake. Until you try it you won't believe how good this cake is—how suave, tender, yet firm, just sweet enough, tasting faintly of lemon beneath the cream.

Don't forget that you can vary this low-calorie cheesecake by serving it with fruit glazes—strawberry, raspberry, peach, etc. Mash fresh fruit, add water and a little lemon juice, sweeten with Sucaryl, thicken with a little cornstarch, and cook lightly. Arrange fresh fruit sections in a pretty pattern on the top of the chilled cheesecake, and pour the glaze carefully over all. Chill.

Lemon Meringue Pie, 110 calories per serving versus 281 calories in traditional recipe.

Lemon Pie Filling, 226 calories versus 1,425 for traditional recipe. Fill measuring cup with water. Empty contents of 2 envelopes of D-Zerta vanilla pudding into small saucepan. Moisten with 1 tablespoon of water from the cup. Add all but a little of the water in the cup. In water remaining, mix 4 tablespoons cornstarch. Gradually add ¾ cup of fresh lemon juice. Add to mixture in saucepan. Cook mixture over medium heat, stirring constantly, until it comes to a boil and thickens. Stir in 1 teaspoon grated lemon peel.

This makes a pungent lemon filling, rather tart. If you like it sweeter, add 1 or 2 Sucaryl tablets before cooking.

Beat 4 egg whites with dash of salt, until stiff. Add cooled filling and stir together until smooth and light.

For crust; Use de-calorized pastry recipe on page 22, pre-baked.

Top with meringue: Beat 2 egg whites, adding 1 teaspoon lemon juice and powdered Sucaryl (about 1 teaspoon) as it thickens. Pile on pie top. Chill. Serves 6.

Quick reference list of the lowest-calorie fruits

These are the fruits to keep on hand:

Low-calorie frozen fruits	*Calories*
½ cup apricots	82
½ cup melon balls	50
½ cup peaches	78
½ cup pineapple	86
½ cup raspberries	98

Low-calorie fresh fruits	
1 medium banana	88
½–⅔ cup pineapple	52
1 cup strawberries	56
(1 berry = 3)	
½ honeydew (5″)	122
½ cantaloupe (4¾″)	60
1 green grape	1
½ cup orange sections	44
¾ cup raspberries	57

9

Make Your Kitchen Diet for You

If you're serious about losing weight or helping someone in your family do it, tackle this project as you would a business problem; or as you'd go about one of your community or club jobs. The theater for this new enterprise is your kitchen. This calls for some retooling, some new staging.

Depend on this: unless your kitchen changes, your measurements won't!

Here's the start that determines the finish

To reorient your cooking, you must first reorient your food shopping. You'll eat what you have in the house. That depends on your shopping list (See Chapter 4 and pages 128–33). Remember to keep only low-calorie foods handy; and you'll lose automatically. But if you don't change your shopping habits, you'll never lose weight for keeps.

Your supply cupboards and refrigerator should be rearranged physically to reflect your new calorie-conscious approach to cooking. Your kitchen bookshelf

117

will carry some new titles. Put your facts about calorie values where you can refer to them often.

Your kitchen utensils and equipment may need replenishing. And please don't underestimate the importance of the role good tools play. As with any other ticklish task, having the right tool at hand when you need it can make the difference between persevering and quitting, between success and failure.

A slapdash attack is almost worse than not starting at all, because discouragement at your inevitable failure tends to send you off on an oh-the-heck-with-it eating binge.

Get set for a long haul

Obviously, shedding pounds that have been years in accumulating isn't going to be done overnight. It's a long-term proposition. And it's a serious one; not a passing fancy, not a matter of vanity, but of health and happiness, even of life and death. Thoughtful organization and helpful equipment will pay you dividends for years in hours of time saved, pounds of weight lost. It's money and brains invested in living. New reducers' helpers will be turning up every few months. Keep an eye peeled for them and add them to your life-prolonging collection.

First, let's consider how the arrangement of your kitchen and how the equipment in it can help shed pounds.

What does your overweight member see when he comes prowling hungrily out to the kitchen making, no doubt, straight for the refrigerator? He should see what he likes, and what's good for what ails him.

How your refrigerator can help

He'll be looking perhaps for something to drink. He should not see whole milk, at 170 calories a glassful. That's tucked back out of sight. In front, is Borden's good new "modified skimmed milk," fat-free, enriched, and vitamin-fortified. Unless of course your reducer likes buttermilk or skimmed milk. Then they are what he sees, naturally. And/or a frosty bottle of tomato juice cocktail, or V-8.

He certainly sees, let us hope, an assortment of chilled sugarless soft drinks in his favorite flavors. These should be the most visible of all drinkables in sight, being the lowest in calories.

What he doesn't see can't tempt him

He undoubtedly is on the prowl for a snack. By no accident, therefore, the most eye-catching thing in the refrigerator is a dish of his favorite raw vegetable bites; crisp white celery and/or carrot sticks or the like. They may be sparkling under a transparent cover of Saran Wrap, but they're all ready to eat. He'll find small fresh fruits, berries in season; a bowl of peaches perhaps, Sucaryl-sweetened, or whatever is his favorite among the excellent dietetic canned fruits. He'll see cold meat loaf, or lean roast; perhaps some hard-boiled (or devilled) eggs; he'll see cottage cheese, Provolone, or his favorite spread.

He doesn't seem to see butter (it's hidden at the back) but he does see a butter dish full of farmer cheese and butter mixed. There are low-calorie jellies; and the same kind of mayonnaise.

Your refrigerator is a key piece

Your refrigerator is a key piece. Is it filled and arranged to help him lose weight? Or is it his daily downfall?

What else does his roving eye catch? Baskets of low-calorie crackers, flat bread, cheese tidbits on the kitchen counter? And if there are cookies in the cookie jar, cake in the cake box, surely they're your own homemade low-calorie kind. Or the low-calorie varieties you can buy, listed on pages 41–42.

If he opens the supply cupboard, what does he see? Package of 20-calorie store-bought cookies; cans of Heinz and Campbell's soup, but only his favorites among the low-calorie varieties.

That supply cupboard of yours holds the secret

of whether or not you really mean it about wanting to see some weight lost in your household. For the items that are now your supply cupboard's solid front, let us look at the brain of your reducing kitchen: your kitchen bulletin board, posted near the telephone, cookbook shelf, and kitchen desk.

How your bulletin board can help

Here we will find, let us hope, a shopping Reminder List; foods you want to be sure you're never short of. (Complete list, pages 128–33.)

Half of Tool No. 1: a calorie-counter

Is your kitchen bulletin board the most strategic place for you to keep a calorie tally? Consult that little book as faithfully as an astrologer consults the stars. Have it within easy reach, with a blackboard or a scratch pad near for your calculations.

Have you discovered how widely calorie-counters vary? Well, they do. Only two are considered authoritative. Pages 170–83 are taken from one: the 147-page USDA's Handbook No. 8; "Composition of Foods." Send to Washington, D.C., for it (free). The other is available from Anna dePlanter Bowes, 7th & Delancey Sts., Philadelphia, Pa.: "Food Values of Portions Commonly Used," 94 packed pages of vital news for $2.25. Vitamin, mineral, cholesterol, and purine content of foods included.

Steep yourself in this twentieth-century witchcraft that will keep you and your husband young and attracted to each other.

Measuring the amount of food is essential to the calorie-counting operation. So you'll need a set of measuring cups and spoons; also a small postal scale* on which the ounce markings are clearly readable. Many calorie calculations that you'll find in the books are in terms of 100 grams; since there are 28 grams to an ounce, this is roughly 3½ ounces. You'll need to weigh meats, cheese, butter, and other concentrations of calo-

---

*Handy for weighing letters, too!

ries at first until your eye has learned calorie quantities.

Only the scale knows the facts; and you'll have some surprises to begin with.

The other half of Tool No. 1

A knowledge of calorie values is basic; just as basic, is a knowledge of the vitality foods.

On pages 128–33 you'll find lists of low-calorie, high-vitality foods that subtract pounds and add sex appeal. On pages 50–55 you discover how and why they work such magic for reducers.

If there are underweights in your family, these are still foods that should be the mainstay of their diet, for health's sake. To put fat on their bones, you have only to add what makes fat; namely pure fat, sweets, starches.

Know the foods that work magic

On page 53 is a list of vitality foods and what they do for you. If you make two copies of the list you can post one on your kitchen bulletin board for reference when you order and assemble meals and keep the other in the drawer of your bedside table, where you can refer to it as you plan what you're going to eat and serve the next day. Looking it over just before you go to sleep will install this vital knowledge in your head more quickly.

How your kitchen bookshelf can help

Your favorite cookbooks will still be your favorite browsing ground no doubt, and now that you're learning how to edit out the hidden calories, they'll take on a new look, present a new challenge. But when you feel an urge to buy a new book, here is a list, all available in paperback, recommended to speed you on to your *bella figura.*

Dr. Atkins' Diet Revolution by Dr. Robert C. Atkins. A Bantam paperback. I "ghosted" this book for Dr. A. I read *hundreds* of case histories, and interviewed *scores* of patients. In two years of this I saw no evidence that this low carbohydrate diet was anything but remarkably effective—and safe. You can disregard all that A.M.A. hullabaloo.

There are just two ways to lose weight besides fasting. One is by eating fewer calories. The other is by cutting your carbohydrate intake way down. This book tells you how to lose by the second method. Those of us who have to fight fat all our lives will probably get around to trying all three methods before we're through. We benefit by the stimulus of a change of approach. A lot of people have lost a lot of weight—and comfortably—with the Dr. Atkins book.

Better Homes and Gardens ® Calorie Counter's Cookbook by the editors of Better Homes and Gardens. Meredith Publishing and Bantam Books.

The Doctor's Quick Weight Loss Diet Cookbook by Irwin M. Stillman, M.D. and Sam Sinclair Baker. A Bantam paperback.

Dr. Atkins' Diet Cookbook by Fran Gare and Helen Monica. A Bantam paperback.

Food Becomes You: Better Health Through Better Nutrition by Ruth M. Leverton. Doubleday.

How your kitchen can help de-calorize meats
Get an electric slicer or at least a good meat carver. Never slice meat thick. Thin slices seem to taste better, anyhow; they look more appetizing, they seem like more, therefore your reducer is content with fewer calories.

Cut bacon's calories up to 200 per cent. One slice of bacon can contain 75 calories. But if you cook your bacon on a bacon crisper, each slice can only be 25 calories, because the fat is scientifically drained off as it cooks. Bacon tastes better too because it cooks more evenly on a bacon crisper.

Plank your fish! Buy one of the handsome wooden baking boards for fish and steak, or cut your own from hardwood. Oak is best. Because fish tastes and looks so infinitely more luxurious with this staging, this best of all calorie protein buys will be welcome more often. Arrange the vegetables around the fish, including the ring of whipped potatoes. This adds to the festive effect and also saves dishwashing.

Broiling happens more often because it's more fun for everybody, including the cook, when it's done with one of the new infra-red, no heat, no smoke, no splatter broilers. And broiling is the reducers' best bet as a meat-cooking method.

A rotisserie is the perfect no-fat way to broil chickens, roasts, spareribs, so that the meat is cooked through: juicy, tender, delectable. And everybody has such a wonderful time superintending the process!

Pretty shell servers for fish concoctions mean that you can serve less and yet have everyone feeling extraordinarily well fed because the fish *looks* so elegant. Adds up to so few calories that you can serve an extra luscious dessert that meal, and still be ahead of the game.

Summer indispensable: a fish mold for those cool, hearty, fish aspics that look almost too pretty to eat and are so wonderfully low in calories.

Low-cost, low-fat meats can quickly be cooked to tender perfection without adding any fat at all, if you have a pressure cooker. A pressure cooker is a wonderful time-and-fat-saver with chicken, stews, ragouts, too. Look for one that is partitioned.

Check list of other meat "musts": Meat thermometer, oven-thermometer, a good roaster and meat rack. Most important of all: a good range!

How your kitchen can help de-calorize eggs

The poached egg, which asks for no butter, is likely to be asked for more often if you have egg poachers to keep the egg neat, and make the process of poaching it as easy and foolproof as boiling water. You can buy Teflon egg-poachers—less work for mother.

Fry eggs or make your omelet in a heavy skillet of cast iron with a permanent porcelainized surface, so pretty it's an ornament to any table. Easy to wash, too, and won't stain or burn out. The merest film of butter is all it requires. If you want puffy omelets, use egg separator and beat whites stiff with rotary or electric beater.

Scramble eggs in a Pyrex double boiler to guarantee perfection every time. Without benefit of butter, too. Pyrex dishes take heat better without fat than most metal cooking dishes. Easy to clean, and moderate in price.

Shirred eggs make a sturdy, delicious low-calorie luncheon or supper dish, with a green salad. Pretty china pottery or copper baking dishes and ramekins keep them piping hot, make them look like more calories than they are. Look for Teflon-lined ones.

Boiling eggs is a fatless procedure and likely to be pushed more frequently in your house if you have a rack or *egg-lifter* to take cooked eggs from boiling water without burning those valued fingers. To guarantee perfect timing on boiled eggs every time get yourself an electric egg cooker. It's automatic; even signals you to come and get them. Get an egg pricker too.

Pretty egg cups will often turn out to be a good reason for having your eggs boiled, too. Why not start collecting a harlequin set of them in antique shops?

Saving calories via vegetables and fruits

Start a collection right now of gadgets and tools that add glamour to those vitamin-packed vegetables and fruits so important to filling up a reducer, while paring him down. These are among the biggest little helps your kitchen has to offer.

For instance:

Get a good melon-baller. Better yet, get 3 good melon-ballers in different sizes. Use them not only to make melon look its most festive and easy to eat, but also to make potato balls—a great potato stretcher, and a mighty pretty dish. Use your melon-baller on cucumbers, too. Tiny fresh cucumber balls in a green salad, an aspic, or alone, with icy yogurt and a sprinkle of parsley, look and taste beautiful. Larger cucumber balls cooked until they're crisp-tender, and fragrant with fresh dill, are a sensation; particularly perfect with fish.

Look for fluted knives, which will cut carrots, cucumbers, and potatoes in thin elegant slices for cooking.

Do you have a sharp grapefruit knife? You'll serve grapefuit more often if you do, because it makes preparing, as well as eating, so much simpler.

How's your supply of vegetable brushes? Good ones, suited to the job in hand, are a must for high-speed food preparation.

Shears for cutting parsley, herbs, and a hundred other jobs are as basic to cooking as to sewing.

A vegetable crisper is a must for reducers. There's a wonderful one called the Tri-State Permacrisp, of chip-proof, feather-light plastic, with a selfseal lid that flips up with a finger tip, and it keeps its contents garden-fresh for an unbelievable length of time.

Be a mold collector because gelatins and aspics make such delectable jewel-cool meals in the summer; salads and desserts all year round. They're rich in protein, rich in vitamins, too. Their beauty and variety permit more frequent serving of those lowest-calorie items: vegetables, fish, fruits. Most kinds can be stored in your freezer, too.

A ring mold and a fruit mold are basics; but you'll lose weight faster if you have a variety of shapes and sizes, because you'll tend to serve gelatins more often. Don't forget, too, how tastily they use up leftovers.

Of course you have a wooden chopping board and one of those talented *Foley* choppers, haven't you? Also a salad bowl and salad servers that you dote on so dearly that you'd like to use them every meal, including breakfast.

Presto-chango slicer-shredder-grater. Beauty treatments for raw vegetables that are low in calories and high in cosmetic results, with the New Enterprise slicer-shredder-grater. Four quick-change cutting discs of stainless steel wash clean in a jiffy. Special pusher lid to press food against blades without endangering your fingers. Carrots come out of it completely transformed, looking like fluffy gold shredded coconut, moist, delicate, delicious in salads. Suction cup feet hold it firm to the table top.

An electric blender is a magician at making dry skimmed milk act, taste, look almost like cream. Add such low-calorie fruits as apricots, or fresh pineapple, fresh peaches or raspberries, then Sucaryl, and the milkshake that machine delivers is nothing short of heavenly.

Its tricks with fresh vegetables are just as inspiring; and it can turn out hollandaise, salad dressings and dessert sauces of incredibly thick creamy richness at a fractional calorie cost, because they start with that smooth deceiver, fresh country cottage cheese, instead of cream or butter.

There's almost nothing this gadget can't do. It's the biggest mechanical help yet devised for reducers . . . bar none! An Osterizer will even make peanut butter! Get one!

A special spatula with a narrow rubber blade that will reach between those blender blades to scrape out every last good drop, is a must. They're made just for this. If you don't find one in your biggest housewares store, send to Macy's, or the nearest big department store.

About dishes. The way to keep a woman quiet, a wise man once said, is to keep her badly dressed.

Conversely, the way to keep you interested in serving vegetables and fruits is to provide yourself with casseroles, plates and serving dishes for them, so charming, so characterful, so expressive of your creative good taste, that you love to use them, to put them on the table, to show them off.

Don't think of these purchases as a luxury, or a self-indulgence. Think of them as a basic tactic by which you're going to achieve a difficult and important end: that of bettering your family's health and happiness, by getting excess weight off them.

Five more ways your kitchen can diet for you

1. *Butter Curler or Butter Paddles.* When butter is molded into small but interesting curls or balls and served individually, less gets eaten than when there's a large plate of it on the table within easy reach. Yet servings somehow don't look stingy when they're so aristocratically decorative.

2. *It Does Matter How You Slice It!* De-calorize cheese with a flick of a slotted knife or chrome or silver plate. The slice it cuts is so tissue-thin that even several slices of that creamy Muenster stay low in calories. The conversation piece of many a cocktail party, and soul-satisfying to operate.

3. *Give Them Waffles More Often.* They're low-budget and luxurious, those waffle suppers and breakfasts. And now that waffles are low-calorie too (see page 20)—*celebrate,* and get one of the new G. E. waffle irons that make four waffles at one whack.

4. *Keep the Pastry Tube Close at Hand*. It stre-e-e-etches the calories in potatoes so that one potato looks like two. And that potato ring dresses up any main dish. For icing, for "whipped cream" toppings, your pastry tube performs the same reducing services; so keep it squeezing.

5. *Stay Serenely Put Through Courses Galore*. No trips to the kitchen needed when you have the help of an electrically heated hot table. The top shelf of radiant glass heats up to keep foods hot; the bottom shelf is of mar-proof formica. Remember: the more courses, the fewer calories!

And if you have one or more of the new mobile serving units—a Cosca tray cart perhaps, or one of those Salton hot tables—a five-course meal actually involves less kitchen trotting than a two-course meal without them.

You probably have some of these cook's helpers already—but perhaps you aren't *using* them. As for those you *don't* have, naturally you can't rush out and get them all—but you can acquire them gradually. Many of them are reasonably inexpensive. In any case, just reading the *list*, will, I hope, give you ideas for extemporizing—and about this new approach to cooking that's long on luxury and short on fat-making calories.

SHOPPER'S CHECK LIST of Low-Calorie Staples for a Reducer's Supply Cupboard

Low-calorie Canned Vegetables

Pumpkin	Pickled Beet Balls
Stewed Tomatoes	Water Chestnuts
Whole Tomatoes	Tiny Brussels Sprouts
Whole Onions	from Holland
Green Asparagus Tips	Bean Sprouts
Sweet and Sour Red	Mushrooms
Cabbage	Bamboo Sprouts
Sauerkraut	Cresca Hearts of Palm
Beets (whole, sliced,	Celeriac (from France)
diced)	

Low-calorie Canned Meats

Bacon
Reese Whole Pheasant
Reese Turkey (in cans)
Reese Breast of Turkey
Reese Partridge
Reese Grouse
Shrimps
Salmon
Lobster
Tuna
Crab Meat
Tiny Boiled Clams

Minced Clams
Sunnam Golden Clams
   in Aspic
Vienna Sausage (only 35
   calories per sausage)
Ox Tongue in Jelly
Dried Beef
Picnic Hams
Sandwich Steaks
Canadian Bacon
Frankfurters

Low-calorie "Starchy" Dishes

Tiny Whole Canned
   Potatoes
Egg Noodles (in all
   shapes)

Progresso Canned Red
   Kidney Beans (cooked
   in salted water)
Pinebridge Farms Canned
   Cooked Wild Rice

Low-calorie Soups

Tomato Aspic
Bouillabaisse
Lobster Stew
Fish Chowder
Bouillon Cubes
Beef Soup
Consommé Cubes
Beef with Vegetables
Turtle Soup
Borsch
Chicken Gumbo
Onion Soup
Gumbo Creole
Black Bean Soup (add
   sherry)

Clam Chowder
Oxtail Soup
Madrilène
Pepper Pot
Chicken Noodle
Bouillon Chicken Rice
Chicken Consommé
Beef Noodle
Vegetable-Beef
Pinesbridge Farms
   Claret Consommé
Pinesbridge Farms Jellied
   Clam Madrilène
Green Pea
Frozen Won-Ton

Most Pickles and Relishes Are Low-calorie

Hot-Dog Relish
Sweet Mixed Pickles
Piccalilli
Mustard Pickles

Dill Pickle
   (spears or sticks)
Cross-cut Pickles
Garlic Olives

Cherry Peppers
Sweet Gherkins
Chow-Chow
Cucumber Pickles
India Relish

Danish Cucumbers
Pickled Beets
Ketchup
Chili Sauce
Reese Tiny Plum Tomatoes

For the Calorie-wise Canapé Shelf

Pumpkin Seeds
Parched Sweet Corn
Sunflower Seeds
Salmon Paste
Lobster Paste
Crab Meat Paste
Shrimp Paste
Smoked Turkey Pâté
Smoked Ham Pâté
Tomato Cocktail Sticks
Celery Onion Sticks
Pretzel Bitz
Onion Flavored Fried
  Bacon Rinds
Cheese Flavored Fried
  Bacon Rinds
Garlic Flavored Fried
  Bacon Rinds
Smoked Sturgeon
Smoked Carp
Whole Smoked Shrimps
Cocktail Sausage
Pâté de foie
Mushrooms in Port Wine
Meat Balls
Cocktail Tamales
Tiny Peeled Shrimps
  in Brine
Sprats
Cocktail Sardines
  in Sherry

Pickled Mushrooms
Anchovy Paste
Artichoke Hearts
Caviar
Tiny Gherkins
Marinated Mussels
Exton Wine Crackers
Peak Frean's Twiglets
Smoked Whitefish
Smoked Salmon
Smoked Eel
Pickled Herring
Gefulte Fish Balls
Tongue Spread
Deviled Ham
Sell's Liver Paste
Sell's Chicken Paste
Cocktail Dumplings
Danish Miniature Fish
  Balls
Crabapple-Smoked Oysters
Corn Kernels
Tiny Dill Tomatoes
Cresca Cocktail Beets
Cocktail Smoked Mussels
Korn Parchies
Cheese Wafer Stix
Devonshire Caratrix
Small Green Olives, with
  pits

Low-calorie Candies (none over 25 calories per piece)

Pascal Buttercup Assort-
  ment (cheap for 4 lbs.,
  5 oz. in a big handsome
  foot-high jar of *good*
  candy)

Life-Savers
Pixie Pops
Charms Spiced Gumdrops
Honey Nougats
Mintees

Court Drops
Fruit Salad
Licorice Satines
Saylor's Coffe-ets
Swiss Raspberries
Cresca Candy Pebbles
(delicious candy that
look *exactly* like little
pebbles; very trick!)
All kinds of Licorice
Mackintosh's Toffee
Wafers
Necco Wafers
Rum and Butter Toffee
English Lemon Sours
English Clear Mints
(made in England)
Old-Fashioned Scotch
Mints

Big Top Lollypops
Michigan Mints
Martinson's Coffee Candy
Mason's Black Crows
Mason's Dots
Mason's Berries
Schutter's Bit O Honey
(small pieces)
Blaney's Molasses Kisses
Jujy Fruits
Flavor Mixture
Martin's Tangerine Drops
English Lime Drops
(made in England)
Bonamo's Turkish Taffy
Good and Plenty
All sour balls

Dairy Products

Cool-Whip (14 calories
per tablespoon)
Golden Sauce
Sta-whip
Whipped Butter
Whipped Nucoa
Instant Dry Skimmed Milk
Cottage Cheese
Pot Cheese
Farmer Cheese
Yogurt
Skimmed Milk
Buttermilk
Cocktail Delight Cheddar
with Port Wine

Cocktail Delight Stilton
with Cherry Brandy
Limburger
Blue Cheese or Roquefort
Kraft and Borden cheese
spreads
Velveeta and other Process
Cheese Foods
Liederkranz
Cheese-Whiz (45 calories
per tablespoon)
Provolone Cheese
Whipped Cream Cheese

Low-calorie Crackers and Toast
(most of these contain 1 to 10 calories per piece)

Mohn Matzos (100 calories
for a whopping 8-inch
square)
Cheese Pretzels
Cheese Cocktailers

Devonshire White Melba
Devonshire Hol-grain
Protein Wafers
Tam-Tam Crackers
Nabisco Oysterettes

Sunshine Cocktail Assortment
Old London Melba Toast and Rounds
Devonshire Melba Rounds
Devonshire Protein Melba
Devonshire Whole Wheat Melba
Devonshire Rye Melba
Bakonets*

Nabisco Pretzel Sticks
Nabisco Triangle Thins
Nabisco Cheese Tidbits
Nabisco Cheddar Cheese Crackers
Norwegian Ideal Flatbread
Finn Thin Crisp Waferettes
Ideal Flatbread

Lower-calorie Cakes and Cookies

Dessert Shells
Wine Loaf
Angel Cake
Sponge Cake
Pound Cake
Marble Pound Cake
Nabisco Wafers
Famous Chocolate Wafers
Nabisco Arrowroot Biscuits
Nabisco Vanilla Wafers
Nabisco Sugar Wafers (small)
Nabisco Ginger Snaps
Nabisco Honey Grahams
Nabisco Chocolate Snaps
FFV Orange Thins
FFV Lemon Thins

Weston Orange Tea Rings
Anise Rusks
Kichel (egg cookies)
Egg Biscuits
Le Fevre Gaufrettes
Le Fevre Biscuits Boudoir
Le Fevre Biscuits Champagne
Huntley & Palmer Afternoon Tea Biscuits
Huntley & Palmer Ginger Brittles
Meringues
Carr's Assorted Cookies
Olibet Petit Beaurre
Olibet Alphabet Cookies
Schmidt-Vienna Patience

Color, Taste, and Texture Dress-ups

Pimento
Black Walnuts (in vacuum-packed tins)
Chocolate Sprinkles
Virginia Dare spangles
Virginia Dare silver Dares
Virginia Dare rubies
Virginia Dare emeralds

Maraschino cherries
Marshmallows
Hazelnuts
Pignolias
Unsalted almonds
Grated Parmesan
Poppy seed
Caraway seeds

*They're fried pork-rinds: light, crisp, delicious—the *only no-carbohydrate crisp* on the market. Look for them under different trade names.

Virginia Dare confetti
Virginia Dare cinnamon
 drops
Shredded Coconut
Candied Ginger
Salted pumpkins
Salted soynuts

Parsley flakes
Capers
Croutons
Garlic croutons
Ice-cream cones
Sesame seeds
Sliced toasted almonds

Good Calorie Buys in the Delicatessen Section

Bologna, per slice
 —66 calories
Liver sausage, per slice
 —79 calories
Luncheon meat, per slice
 —81 calories
Lean roast beef
Cold tongue

Cold corned beef
Canadian bacon
Fresh sauerkraut
Beet salad
Coleslaw
Cold turkey
Cold chicken
Lean boiled ham

Low-calorie Frozen Foods for Your Home Freezer

Melon balls
Cod fillets
Halibut steaks
Sole fillets
Scallops
Oysters
Flounder fillets
Ocean perch fillets
Rock lobster tails
Mountain trout
Crab meat
Veal cutlets
Calves' liver
Pork chops
Whipped potatoes
Squash

Green beans
Shrimps
Lobster
Chicken breasts
Chicken livers
Sandwich steaks
Broccoli
Brussels sprouts
Spinach
Asparagus
Minute Maid unsweetened,
 fresh pineapple juice
Minute Maid fresh frozen
 grapefruit sections
Ice-milk frozen dessert
Artichoke hearts

Reminder: In the dietetic food section, order these youth-savers *by the case:* fruits in sweet, heavy, no-calorie syrup (I like the Diet-Sweet brand best): Dorset Diet-Pack Tomato Soup and their Mushroom Soup; D-Zerta gelatin desserts, and new sugar-free D-Zerta puddings; Choc-Low. Make up a list from Chapter 4.

Note: Some de-calorized foods aren't always in the dietetic food section, but mixed with regular brands; the de-calorized soft drinks, for example.

Important: If you don't find what you want ASK THE MANAGER. If he doesn't stock it, ASK HIM TO! Remember what stores stock depends *entirely* on what customers want.

Don't give up if he's uninterested. Bring this book along next time and show it to him. Keep pleasant and perhaps *next* time you ask, half a dozen other people will have asked too; and the manager will have changed his mind.

Don't be a rabbit; this is important to you; throw your weight around politely. This trend to low-calorie foods has revolutionized the food and drink industry. *Remember, 3 out of 4 Americans worry about how much they weigh.* What you want, MOST people want. You can get it.

Here are some names and addresses to give your grocer to *keep after him* with!

Diet Delight products, California Canners and Growers Association, 3100 Ferry Building, San Francisco, California.

Dietician Foods (for Choc-Low etc.), 311 King's Highway, Orange, New Jersey.

Tillie Lewis Foods Inc., Stockton, California 95201.

The Pillsbury Co., Pillsbury Building, Minneapolis, Minn.

Betty Crocker (for the homogenized pie-crust sticks), General Mills, 9200 Wayzata Blvd., P.O. Box 1113, Minneapolis, Minn.

10

Fooling Those Alcohol Calories

If you have to lose a lot of weight fast you'll avoid all alcohol religiously. Nothing has more calories than alcohol, except fat itself. Sixteen hundred calories in a pint of whisky, in case you think you want to drink a pint at a sitting.

And alcohol provides no dietary essentials except energy. Don't be cheered by any loose talk you hear that alcohol calories can't be stored in the body as fat. They can't, it's true. But that doesn't help you a bit. Alcohol does contain calories. So you have to add your alcohol calories in with the rest, just as if they were food calories. There is a reason: if the total number of calories you eat and drink in a day exceeds the number you burn up, your body uses the alcohol calories for energy and stores the excess food calories as fat.

Doctors differ

A few years ago not one doctor in a thousand would have allowed for a cocktail in the reducing diet he prescribed. A lot of them still won't hear of it.

"With the food intake drastically curtailed to lower calorie-intake, every item on the diet must make an important nutritional contribution," these diet-hards maintain quite logically.

No doctor quarrels with this theory. "The trouble

is it only works when the dieters are rats," a doctor I know observed wryly.

The result of years of dealing with dieters who are convivial, highly fallible human beings has wrought great changes since the naïve old days when overweight was treated as a simple nutritional disorder. *The New York Times* reports Dr. David B. Hand as warning a convention of nutritionists, "Don't take the fun out of eating. A diet that's a grim business won't work."

But many "allow" alcohol

An increasing number of doctors permit a cocktail, a highball, or a few glasses of beer with the diets they prescribe for patients who are not too drastically overweight.

This is in line with the new realization that the only solution to your overweight is an eating program you can live with the rest of your life; one that keeps the calories down, yet is flexible enough to fit the year-in and year-out pattern of your days. So, unless you're a teetotaler, or a hermit, you've got the problem of doing a certain amount of business and/or social drinking while still keeping a flat middle. What are the best strategies?

Know alcohol calories

Strategy number one is to know your alcohol calories. Here they are, per ounce. Of course you seldom drink so strictly by the ounce. But this gives you a comparative notion as to the concentration of alcohol calories in the various drinks you usually have to choose from. (The higher the proof, the higher the calories.)

	calories per ounce		*calories per ounce*
vodka, 80-proof	80	champagne, dry	24
gin	72	French vermouth,	
scotch	72	dry	30
bourbon	90	Italian vermouth,	
rye	78	sweet	48
Bacardi	70	red wine, dry	20
cognac	75	white wine	
cordials	70	(sauterns)	24
port	45	beer	12
sherry, dry	40		

Strategy number two is to count those calories.
Have the house littered with jiggers, if necessary. But be
sure there's always a one-ounce jigger, and a one and a
half-ounce jigger anywhere there's a bottle in your
household.

And keep counting! There's a universal tendency
to stop counting when you stop feeling virtuous and
begin to feel guilty over how many you've had.

You're safe—as long as you can count

But there's a mystic virtue in keeping count. As
long as you keep count you're still on top of the whole
project.

To help you count, here's approximately how highballs made with soda or water turn out.

If you make them with ginger ale or tonic water
you must add 100 calories per glass. But why not use
sugarless drinks as your mixer, in which the calories
are so few that you needn't count them at all?

highballs:	1½ -ounce jigger, with soda or water
scotch	108
bourbon	135
rye	118
brandy	112

As for cocktails, these vary so much depending
on how much ice is used, how much of it has melted
into the drink, the size of the glass, the amount of
vermouth or other more dilute ingredients, that you'll
do well to add up the calories yourself, jigger by jigger,
as you make the mix.

Don't try to change your spots

If nothing but a cocktail gives you the lift you like,
then accept the fact. As long as you count those cocktail
calories in your day's score, you can still keep those calories down, and live it up modestly.

If you're the flexible type and can tolerate any
change in the sacred ritual at all, you might take up
martinis, manhattans, etc., on the rocks.

This trend toward cocktails on the rocks seems to have grown less out of calorie-consciousness than out of a wholesome caution as to what a late dinner hour and too many cocktails before can do. People who have grown attached to the custom also claim they like the fact that the ice keeps the mixture properly frosty. Certainly a warm cocktail is no gourmet's dish.

Discover spritzers

If you like wine, the low-calorie way to drink it is the way they do it by the banks of the blue Danube, in a spritzer: a "highball" of dry white wine and soda. A spritzer is cool, light, and pleasant anytime. It's especially refreshing in summer and has considerably fewer calories than a whisky highball. But count the jiggers of wine that go in. Twenty-five calories per ounce-jigger, remember?

Extremely pleasant in a low-watt way is the lowest calorie gambit of all: a jigger of dry vermouth and soda in a tall glass or an Old-Fashioned glass, with a twist of lemon peel; only 30 calories for this. And you can dawdle with it indefinitely, filling it up with soda when it's half gone. It has a clean woodsy taste and fragrance; light, but there's a little lift in it too.

Yes, *Slimming* Sangria

I learned to make a quick-easy sangria in London from some young hard-up artists; 3 parts of cheap red Spanish wine and 2 parts of Schweppes Tonic Water, with slices of lemon and orange. Surprisingly good, but *not* slimming. (Many people have the delusion that regular Tonic Water is non-calorific. Wrong. Just as many calories as colas or any other sugar-sweetened drink.) However, back in America, I make it with No-Cal Tonic water (½ a calorie to the ounce). And I make it half and half so a *pitcherful*—with red wine only costing 20 calories per ounce and with the displacement of ice and fruit slices—doesn't come to more than two or three hundred calories. One hot day, try it; what can you lose?

Luckily, most everybody likes beer

Newly chic, and just the opposite of esoteric, is beer, America's favorite alcoholic beverage.

Now I know that beer has always been considered the most fattening thing you can put in your mouth. The ads tried to tell us different for a while. But they did in a strangely unconvincing way. They talked about less starch and less sugar, less filling, and more weight-reduced, and more calorie-controlled. It just sounds like more advertising double-talk. A hoax.

Why doesn't the beer industry just tell the truth, the whole truth and nothing but the truth? Beer contains about 100 calories per 8-ounce glass. And the new "light-weight" beers (which means de-carbohydrated) contain 30% fewer calories. Don't knock them until you've tried them. They're light—like Mexican beer. Most of my friends have grown to prefer them to the heavier, sweeter traditional beers.

Because a social soul's toughest problem is likely to be alcohol calories, and because beer is such a godsend in defending a reducer from some of his worst enemies, I think this ubiquitous drink is worth a chapter all to itself.

11

How Beer Can Help You Lose Weight

First, let's get straight on this matter of exactly how fattening beer is. I was so sure that beer must be high calorie that I made a special project of getting its calorie count via the august firm of Bull & Roberts, food chemists, and via oxygen bomb calorimetry. I stood around and watched while Bull & Roberts put two bottles of beer through the calorimeter. One brand we tested contained 100.4 calories per 8 ounces. The other brand tested contained 92.8 calories per 8-ounce glass. (The de-carbohydrated beers, remember, contain 30% *less!*)

The beer-is-fattening myth

So I was wrong, because that's a lot of drinking for around 100 calories or 67 calories if it's a de-carbohydrated brand.

The Germans used to call beer "liquid bread" and they weren't so far wrong. Traditional beer is made of yeast and grains, like bread, and contains 2.2 grams of protein. A slice of bread contains from 1.4 to 2 grams of protein.

Beer has other nutrients too; three times as much riboflavin, almost as much calcium, more niacin than any slice of bread. Its nutritive value is about the same as that of those much-touted breakfast cereals that are supposed to make supermen out of small boys after one box.

Not that all this is any particular reason for drinking beer. You can get far more nutrition for your calories than in beer. But still, what health values you get are pure velvet. If you like beer . . . it would be hard to take your two grams of protein and your 108 micrograms of riboflavin more congenially than in a cool bottle of sparkling beer.

Your no. I hazard: the social drink

If beer's your favorite drink, and you're trying to lose weight, you're lucky. Because your favorite drink, taken in moderation, defends you against the number one hazard of all reducers: the social drink.

Sticking with beer can make a lot of difference in your calorie intake when you go out to cocktail parties. Or out for a big gala evening that lasts until the wee hours. Or during those long public relations lunches, over which so much of the nation's business gets done.

There are three reasons why saying "I'd like beer, please" can help you lose weight.

Reason one: beer fills you up more than other alcoholic drinks.

Reason two: you can make your beer last without being conspicuous about it. When there's a partly filled bottle in front of you, you aren't so likely to be harried by hosts or ebullient companions to "Have another drink, do!" A gesture at your bottle usually quiets the commotion.

Reason three: you know exactly how many calories you're taking in, per bottle—150, or a few less. Result: you aren't as likely to cheat on yourself, as when liquor is sloshed carelessly into a cocktail shaker or your highball glass.

Alcohol mobilizes your "won't power"

Those murderous alcohol calories add up in a very sneaky way. They're terrifyingly high-calorie. But, even more dangerous, they make you feel, "Aw, who cares —so I'm fat! What of it! I've got to have *some* fun! Just this once," etc., etc.

But beer is only 3.6 per cent alcohol. To get the alcohol in one fair-sized martini, you'd have to drink around a full quart of beer.

Because beer has so little alcohol and so much food in it, comparatively, those well-known higher nerve centers aren't so quickly anesthetized. If you take beer, you can live a normal social life, and still stay on top of your calorie intake and your long-range objective about losing weight. And few drinks can give quite the feeling of relaxed well-being that beer gives.

Hazard no. 2: the bedtime snack

If the social drink is a reducer's number one hazard, the bedtime snack is likely to be number one runner-up.

But the average man, at least, will take a bottle of beer for a nightcap, and feel he's well off. Even with a 30-calorie handful of those little pretzel sticks or cocktail crackers, this is a much better calorie buy than a glass of milk and the sandwich and cake that's so likely to insinuate itself along with the milk. The latter combination runs up to 500 to 800 calories, as compared to a bottle of traditional beer's 150 calories. And beer is solidly conducive to a good night's sleep. "Better than a sleeping pill," one doctor wrote in a learned treatise on beer's remarkable powers for soothing and uplifting the human spirit.

Lupulin and tannin are the elements in beer that are credited with the euphoria it produces. Pharmaceutically treasured since doctors wore witch paint, they make beer simultaneously a sedative and a tonic, a combination no hard-pressed modern is going to fight against.

From saloons to salons

It's a nice thing for weight-watchers that beer's social status has risen since women have taken over the buying of the family beer (and a good deal of its drinking, too).

The mugs and steins that were customary when beer was the American workingman's drink are rapidly disappearing as beer has acquired a new cachet typical of today's whole trend toward unpretentious, informal, good living.

Beer has undoubtedly come out of the saloons and into the salons also because it's a gourmet's choice as accompaniment for some of our most upstage dishes: lobster, shrimp, oysters, all sea food, in fact. Clementine Paddleford noted recently that no wine can compete with curry's spiciness; beer's cool, sharp freshness is called for.

Beer goes with today's young living

Whatever the reasons, most people nowadays serve beer and ask for beer any old time. The glasses beer is served in are as formal and elegant as anything else served as a beverage.

Emily Post, of course, always has specified goblets for table beer. They hold six ounces and are of the same delicacy as good wine glasses. They make your beer last and last, because you get three good glasses out of your bottle, allowing room for its head.

However, these informal days most women feel they don't need any more authority than their own sense of style to serve anything in anything. And since mankind has been drinking beer for some seven thousand years, you could find plenty of precedent for serving beer in anything you choose, from brandy inhalers to eyecups.

Champagne glasses are special

It was theater people who started the fashion of serving beer in small, tall glasses. At any rate, you see beer served surprisingly often these days in champagne glasses. It seems to have begun at the 21 Club. Mac Kriendler doesn't remember exactly when and who started it. Anyhow, his stage and screen patrons (whose incomes depend on keeping their figures) have taken it up mightily. Well, it allows them to drink, be social, yet watch their calories. A bottle of beer sipped from a champagne glass lasts easily through the meal, and you've absorbed only 100 (or/150 calories instead of the 400 or 500 calories a couple of 21's nice big dry martinis cost).

If we were calorie-counting robots, or if we lived in a vacuum, or if we would devote our lives to our figures, we wouldn't eat or drink anything except what was on the doctor's diet list. As things are, however, what you drink must be a nice compromise you work out yourself, based on what you like best to drink that costs the least calories.

If you like straight whisky with soda or water better than a cocktail, you're lucky. If you like beer a lot you've even luckier. It's low in alcohol content, and therefore in calories. Its bubbly tang is a soul mate to practically all our favorite dishes. It makes people happy, relaxed, and affectionate. And it doesn't cost much, praise the Lord.

12

How Your Husband Can Lose Weight Without Dieting

Most women feel it's nice to have a man around the house. Especially if he's feeling good. However, if you don't agree, there's a nice legal way to kill your husband off—just feed him to death. It may take some time, but it's sure, sure as shooting.

The trouble is that these overstuffed husbands aren't always obliging enough to pop off immediately. They can blow up in stages. A stroke, or any one of a dozen concomitants of overfeeding makes them chronic invalids, unable to work or make love or enjoy life. Any doctor or insurance man can give you hair-raising figures that show how your husband's excess pounds can mean your having to learn early to live alone and like it.

In an article by Dr. Louis I. Dublin in the *Reader's Digest,* entitled "Stop Killing Your Husband," we learn that "between 70 per cent and 80 per cent more men die in their early fifties usually from some form of heart or circulatory disease largely contributed to by overweight."

Was Shakespeare omniscient? More than three hundred years ago he wrote, "Make less thy body hence; know that the grave doth gape for thee *thrice* wider than for other men."

145

Futures aside, a flat man is more fun to have around right now than a fat man. He's more likely to stay awake after dinner, and he's more likely to be interested in going places and doing things.

Flat men are more interested in women; fat men are more interested in eating and dozing. Flat men aren't as allergic to swimming trunks or dance music as fat men are. Flat men make more money than fat men, whose reactions in business, as at home, are likely to be lethargic most of the afternoon.

In helping your husband to lose weight without trying, your strategy is threefold.

1. GET SET—AND THEN KEEP TRACK

Obviously, your husband's weight reduction program must start with his co-operation and approval. How you cut his calories he'll leave to you. Especially if you can arrange to let him have his cake and keep his figure! But to get under way he has to start with the wind behind him.

First comes a trip to the doctor,* so you both know the poundage you're aiming for, among other useful things. This visit will probably leave your husband wiser, sadder, and mobilized to do something about those excess pounds. He's likely to leave the doctor in an open-minded and curious mood as to what's what in calorie values. Now is a good time to ask him to drop in at a bookstore and pick up a vest-pocket-sized calorie counter that he can take out to lunch with him. This will help him pick his favorites off the restaurant menu at lunchtime, and still make good calorie buys.

While facts about food are operationally in your department, any facts that he's interested in learning for himself will help protect him from at least the mistakes of ignorance.

---

*Ask him about the new, less bothersome, far more accurate P.B.I. metabolism test.

Little black book

It adds a sporting interest to this whole project if you keep a private case history on your private patient. It's a wise precaution, for the first few months at least, to keep track not only of his weekly weight but of the calorie count of the breakfasts and dinners you feed him. Then you can either increase or cut down their caloric value, depending on how the patient progresses.

This case history will encourage both of you as he loses, and gets fitter and fitter instead of fatter and fatter. Call attention to his progress, as you note it in the book. I needn't tell you how a bit of flattery charges a reducer's battery, and actually speeds progress.

Be relaxed

Warning: Don't let your interest betray you into exerting any pressure on your husband to cut down on his food fun. If reducing becomes an issue and there's tension on the subject, you'll run into passive resistance, suspicion, and perhaps open revolt. Putting the arm on him conversationally will hinder rather than help. Making cracks about what he eats can't reach target anyhow. As Cato the Censor told those Romans who were clamoring for an extra ration of grain, "It is a difficult task, my friends, to speak to the belly, because it hath no ears."

2. DON'T SPARE THE AMMUNITION

The cleverer you are, the higher the charge of proteins, vitamins, and minerals you'll be able to smuggle into your husband's calories, to keep him in good health and good humor. Stoke him up on proteins particularly. It's easy; they're man's favorite type of fodder: meats, eggs, cheese, fish. Solidly filling, proteins satisfy the appetite earlier, make it content to use fewer calories. Also proteins step up his metabolism (which, like yours, slows down after 40).

The doctor will probably prescribe supplementary vitamin pills, and perhaps protein and mineral supplements, too. In these days of hydrogenated oils, refined flours, and generally overprocessed and undervitalized foods, a vitamin supplement is a wise health insurance, whether you're underweight, overweight, or an ideal weight. But you still need all you can get in your regular meals.

A juggling act that pays off

So you start juggling: nutrient ammunition, calories, and his food favorites; plus, of course, the ever-present food budget. It's a lot easier than balancing your checkbook, and because it presents a challenge, it isn't a chore.

Nutritional musts

Four groups of nutrients are essential daily.
They are listed here with some sources. Some
foods give more than one essential.

1. Protein—skimmed milk products, eggs, meat, fish.
2. Vitamin C—citrus fruits, tomatoes, raw cabbage.
3. B vitamins—skimmed milk products, yeast, liver.
4. Calcium and iron—molasses, milk, eggs, vegetables of cabbage family.

PROCEED WITH CAUTION: LET YOUR HUSBAND BE YOUR GUIDE

In cooking as in dancing, the better you follow his lead, the more pleasure you get. This is a fact wives usually discover early. So in relieving your husband of that excess baggage he carries around his middle, all your cues must come from him.

If he's going to lose weight and like it, obviously it's got to be done with his favorite dishes. Your fell purpose is to choose from among his favorite dishes those that are either low-calorie to begin with, or can be substantially de-calorized. This gives you lots of latitude, because almost any recipe will yield hidden calories if you approach the problem creatively. But there are a few poisons that you would do well to keep out of the house. Potato chips, for instance. Hard sauce. Doughnuts.

Book his favorites

You start by making a list of your husband's favorite foods. You may say, "That's silly. I know them as well as I know my own."

That's undoubtedly true—but do you give *yourself* any great variety of the things you like? How often have you gone out to a friend's, or to a new restaurant, had something you've always loved and said to yourself, "Gracious, I haven't had this for years. And I adore it. I must remember to have it at home."

Think back to your courting days. Get him to talking about the food of his youth. And about the things he had on vacation trips that tasted so wonderful. Unobtrusively, "research" him as if you were a writer for *The New Yorker* getting material for a profile. Anybody will talk about food.

Is he a big eater?

A big eater is usually a fast eater. And food bolters tend to wash their food down with a glass or more of liquid. You'll pick up some tricks to combat this disease (supposed to be peculiarly American) elsewhere in this book. Such as dividing the meal into many courses, "forgetting" the water, etc.

But if he's a big eater, make the meals look as big as possible. You do this by concentrating on the big-scale vegetables; like broccoli, asparagus, big baked potatoes. You cook the carrots whole. A quartered cabbage looks a whale of a lot bigger than the same number of calories' worth of creamed spinach, or *petit pois*. Concentrate, too, on meats that look big because they have a lot of bone: bone-filled roasts and steaks and chops; shellfish served in the shell; whole roasted chicken, turkey.

Use big plates and spread the food out so the plates look lavishly filled. A variety of vegetables helps with this optical illusion. Make the table look filled with assorted low-calorie side dishes and kickshaws like pickles, relishes, finger salad, etc.

But it takes more than psychology to satisfy a big eater. He's not going to stop eating until he feels solidly full up, satiated. Some foods have far more satiety value than others. These are the foods that linger longer in the stomach and intestines. Also one feels satiated more quickly when the food requires considerable chewing, when one's teeth are given a lot to do, so that the experience of eating is prolonged and pleasantly effortful. Finally, sweets have great satiety value. That's why most people feel that a dinner without dessert is less satisfying than a dinner with dessert.

Clinical tests prove that meats and sweets have the highest satiety value. Next, come milk and milk products, and cooked eggs. Scrambled and hard-boiled eggs have greater satiety value than raw eggs, for the simple reason that they take longer to digest. It may surprise you to hear that soft bread and potatoes, which go quickly down the gullet and pass quickly through the intestines, have little satiety value.

So to keep your big eater happy, give him big foods to feast his eyes on, but give him big solid foods, too, like lots of lean meat, and eggs and milk products. And for dessert, perhaps cheese along with a sweet fresh apple; or one of your big flashy low-calorie desserts, just as sweet as he can take it. No calories in Sucaryl, so why not?

Is he a bedtime snacker?

What of it, when your cakes and pies are only around 100 calories a hunk, the milk he finds in the refrigerator is either fat-free or a low-calorie mixture, when beer is only 100 or 150 calories a bottle? He can't do himself too much damage. This bedtime snack will usually be determined by what he finds in the refrigerator—and the goddess in charge can have that well in hand.

Of course, if he has a tendency to sneak in practically the big meal of the day at bedtime, you may have to spoil him a little. Like offering to bring him a tray with some of those snack suggestions you'll see on pages 118 and 119. It's a certain amount of trouble but it's going to make you look awfully good—and it will get *you* in nice young shape too. *All* over-weight people are big night-time eaters. That's their downfall time.

Is he something of a chef himself?

Get him to do the de-calorizing—*and* the cooking. The more you hand him the ball, the more interested he'll be, and the faster he'll lose. It is as important to his self-esteem to look well in a bathing suit, as it is to yours. He'll probably be just as interested as you are in this de-calorizing business. If you can do the whole thing together, it will be a lot more fun.

Exercise does help—both of you!

So much has been made of the fact that nobody is likely to lose weight permanently by exercise alone, that the helpfulness of exercise in a look-younger program has tended to be ignored. Here again it's the psychological effects added to the physiological effects that do the business. The more overweight one gets, the more passive one tends to become. Which is chicken and which is egg doesn't matter. The point is, fat and bodily stodginess add up to an effect of age and unattractiveness.

Dr. Jean Mayer and his colleagues in Harvard's Nutrition Department have proved by a series of studies that exercise permits you to eat more, without gaining; and that it *doesn't* increase the average person's appetite. Another old wives' tale bites the dust!

No one thing does as much to keep one young, as moving about briskly, frequently, and habitually. It's what keeps us pliant and juicy: keeps pink in the cheek and spark in the eye; it gives tone to the functioning of our lungs, lights, and liver, as well as to our outlook on life.

The one-two-three, bend-stretch-stoop type of calisthenics may do the job physically, and a fine thing, if you're one of those who can stay with this rather joyless activity. But walks, golf, tennis, swimming, bowling, skiing, ping-pong, ice-skating are best because, in these tense and harried days, they give your nervous system badly needed time off.

Take some dancing lessons with him. There's nothing like this kind of honest, innocent fun to keep you both young, happy, attractive, and functioning on all levels at the top of your efficiency. Give Eros—and the life instincts—a break, with this easy, do-it-yourself therapy. The mere sight of yourself in those full-length mirrors improves your posture, provides a potent new incentive for shedding pounds. Come winter it's extra hard to wangle exercise; yet this is when we need it most. If you're clever, you'll use this fact as a persuader to get yourself and spouse signed up for a nice long expensive session at a dancing school. And there's probably nothing as good for what ails most of us, come January, and the onset of years, pounds, and deadening routine. Unless of course you can take six weeks' vacation together somewhere in the sun.

If your husband has a favorite sport, or sports, never stop trying to get him to revive them. And keep exploring until you discover how he can complement them with others, so that there's something he likes to do all the year round. There's a book called *The Encyclopedia of Games* that you might look at, in your library. Just to inspire both of you.

Does he come home from the office starved?

Have edibles on display all over the house. They're as much a part of an attractive home, anyhow, as flowers or greens that delight the eye, comfortable chairs, cheerful lighting. A big bowl of apples, or whatever fruit is in season; apothecary jars full of low-calorie candy (see page 41); a bowl of nuts in the shell; a basket of pretzel sticks, cheese tidbits, or some other low-calorie nibble; at cocktail time: celery, carrot sticks, etc. (See suggestions on pages 129–31.)

Overweights are very likely to be nibblers. You can't change this habit without making them unhappy; you can give them the illusion they're not dieting by letting them continue to nibble low-calorie snacks.

An eating pattern he can lose on . . .

Take a look at the menus on the following pages for a week of cold-weather meals and a week of hot-weather meals. These are strictly fanciful weeks, since in practical fact you'd probably be serving the left-overs of some of those chickens and roasts, instead of starting from scratch every day.

Also, this is rather a heavy succession of meals; perhaps a bit more dinner than you normally serve seven days in a row. But it helps the illusion you're trying to foster. It keeps him from thinking of himself as being on a diet. And the sooner he forgets to remember that he's supposed to be dieting, and just enjoys the good food you give him, the more likely he is to stay on an even keel of normal intake.

Here is an eating pattern he can reduce on . . . *and live with forever.*

Weekday breakfast: around 400 calories.
Restaurant lunch (using his pocket calorie counter as guide): 600 calories including whisky or a bottle of beer.
Cocktail time (whisky or bottle of beer before dinner, and bites to go with them): 250 calories.
Dinner (see 14 sample menus at the end of the chapter): around 700 calories.
Bedtime snack: 150 calories.
Total: around 2,100 calories.

If he's at all overweight the chances are that this is anywhere between 1,000 and 2,500 calories less a day than he's been taking in; and 500 to 1,500 less calories than he's likely to burn up in a day. This much calorie "saving" will cause him to ease off between one and three pounds a week, even allowing for occasional orgies.

Because he's losing one to three pounds a week without dieting, he keeps right on losing, week after week after week, sometimes faster, sometimes slower, but steadily sloughing off the flab, every day a few ounces—thanks, madam, to you. This puts him way ahead of a ten-day wonder diet, which may get flashy results for ten days, but leaves him right where it found him in ten weeks. When it comes to achieving one's ideal weight and keeping that way, this long way around is the only way home, not just the shortest, but positively the only entrance.

Cold-Weather Dinners

	De-calorized Calories Per Serving	Calories Per Serving Traditional Recipes
SUNDAY		
½ grapefruit, broiled with sherry	75	75
*duck à l'orange	200	300
*broccoli with hollandaise sauce	94	225
whipped potatoes	75	100
endive, Roquefort dressing	50	125
hot French bread, butter	100	125
*Boston cream pie	96	290
	690	1240
MONDAY		
clams on the half shell	75	75
*corned beef and cabbage	375	625
boiled potato	85	85
sliced tomatoes, with chopped green pepper	40	40
rye bread, butter	100	100
*pumpkin pie	100	263
	775	1188
TUESDAY		
onion soup, croutons, Parmesan cheese	70	70
*roast chicken or turkey, stuffing	235	450
*cranberry sauce	24	139
*pseudo-sweet potato fluff	80	300
green peas and mushrooms	65	95
*2 hot muffins, butter	92	280
chocolate éclair	170	320
	736	1654

	De-calorized Calories Per Serving	Calories Per Serving Traditional Recipes
WEDNESDAY		
cream of mushroom soup	44	143
*roast beef hash	300	500
buttered green beans	60	60
*sweet-corn pudding	94	250
*salad greens, Russian dressing	50	110
*apple pie	123	331
	671	1394
THURSDAY		
broiled rock lobster tails	100	100
*asparagus with hollandaise sauce	99	230
*chow mein or chop suey	275	325
rice	75	75
*2 slices buttered toast	80	160
*lemon meringue pie	110	281
	739	1171
FRIDAY		
Heinz pea soup with frankfurter "pennies"	85	85
planked fish with potato border	180	280
broiled tomatoes, parsley topped	40	40
*cheese-stuffed green pepper	70	200
*chocolate layer cake	117	350
*ice cream	45	147
	537	1102
SATURDAY		
½ cantaloupe	30	30
lettuce wedges with cucumber dressing	50	100
*cheese soufflé with diced ham	75	140
*scalloped tomatoes	200	410
*fruit sherbet with frosted cake square	200	450
	555	1130

Hot-Weather Dinners

	De-calorized Calories Per Serving	Calories Per Serving Traditional Recipes
SUNDAY		
shrimps with cocktail sauce	50	75
*hot or cold chicken in a basket	115	235
*au gratin potatoes	100	225
cold asparagus vinaigrette	40	75
*2 blueberry muffins, butter	100	288
peaches and "whipped cream"	100	150
*chocolate cup cake with fluffy white icing	70	220
	575	1268
MONDAY		
jellied madrilène	25	25
scallions, radishes, celery, cherry tomatoes	60	60
2 hamburgers (ground lean meat)	300	500
*potato salad	100	180
2 slices buttered toast**	80	160
*ice-cream cake, with butterscotch cake	138	420
	703	1345
TUESDAY		
antipasto	100	200
tossed greens, French dressing	50	125
*spaghetti and meat sauce, Parmesan cheese	256	500
hot garlic bread, buttered	130	130
*lemon ice	22	177
*brownie	70	250
	628	1382

	De-calorized Calories Per Serving	Calories Per Serving Traditional Recipes
WEDNESDAY		
honeydew melon with prosciutto ham	100	100
*tuna casserole, with toast points**	153	297
string-bean salad	55	105
corn on cob	125	125
*coconut snowball, chocolate sauce	125	290
	558	917
THURSDAY		
fruit cup	75	75
*green salad, Roquefort dressing	75	150
*veal curry with rice	240	410
chutnies, ground peanuts, coconut, etc.	100	100
*2 hot muffins, butter	92	280
*ice-cream sundae, chocolate sauce	70	227
*date-and-nut bar	80	260
	732	1502
FRIDAY		
oysters on half shell	100	100
whole cold lobster, with mayonnaise, hard-boiled egg and tomato wedges, olives, coleslaw, breadsticks, butter	350	600
	100	100
*blueberry pie à la mode	118	451
	668	1251

Asterisks indicate that low-calorie recipes for these dishes are given elsewhere in this book.

13

How to Help Yourself Lose Weight

FIVE SPEEDER-UPPERS AND A TWO-DAY "DIET TREAT" THAT WILL TAKE OFF TWO TO FIVE POUNDS

The same de-calorized cooking that enables your family to lose weight without conscious effort, is also going to take the pounds off you. But you have special difficulties too—just as your husband has—and your youngster.

You're the one who has to spend more time in the kitchen hovering over food than anyone else in the house. You have more temptations to eat, because you have more opportunities. When you get the urge to eat your head off, or to take a quick high-calorie snack —because you're hungry, or tired, or bored, or mad, or sad—there's no beneficent goddess to edit the calories out of your food before you're exposed to it. Fortunately you're in a position to help yourself cope with your temptations as no one else can. You can even help yourself to lose weight more quickly than the others. You can lead the parade.

To begin with, you're the expert. You know your way around the low-calorie food field better than anyone else in the family. You always know what you're eating. Most eating mistakes are the result of folly plus ignorance. Yours will just be the result of folly!

158

That's bound to cut down considerably on the number of eating mistakes one makes.

Secondly, you can very well oversee your own weight reduction program with more continuity and authority than you can oversee anyone else's program. And that's important.

Besides what you eat, there's how fast you eat, how often you eat, how stylishly you eat, how consciously you eat. All these might be called the dynamic factors, as distinguished from the mechanical factors in weight reduction.

Here are five basic strategies for helping you to speed the process of dropping pounds; five strategies that take your special temptations into account, too. Only at first you will have to practice these five strategies consciously:

Strategy I

Count your calories—in writing. This calls for three props: A small scale which you keep in the kitchen and use for weighing your portions of food. You'll want to be able to read the ounce markings easily, also the half-ounce markings.

A complete calorie counter, so that you can check the calorie value of each portion of every food and drink.

A calorie calendar. Get a standard desk calendar and each day write down what you ate and drank, how much, and the caloric value of each item. Note the total each day. Average the daily totals at the end of the week, when you weigh yourself.

As long as you count your calories, you'll lose. This device works subtly to keep you conscious of your intake—and that's half the battle. Also, it keeps your unconscious mind "on the ball" so that inner resistances are conspicuous only by their absence.

Only by counting your calories can you learn

the calorie values of different foods. It's a bit like learning a foreign language. And this is the daily lesson that in time makes you master of this information, so vital to your job of guarding the waistlines —and life lines—of your husband and family. Not to mention your own sex appeal.

There's only one way to count calories; write down everything you eat as soon as possible after you eat it, also it's amount and its calorie value. Only in this way can you keep an accurate tally. And the writing down helps enormously to install the knowledge in your mind, for keeps. Also, it shows you your own eating pattern.

Strategy 2

> *Plan your next day's eating* just before you go to sleep. And write it down. Keep a pad and pencil by your bed for this. Or note it on your calorie calendar.

First, think over what you'll be doing next day. Then plan what you'll eat to fit in that particular day's schedule. Three meals—and include two or three between-meal meals. Be ingenious about giving yourself what you like best to eat, while keeping the calorie count low. Write down the calorie value of each portion, and calculate the total in advance.

Don't think first of what is low-calorie. *Think first of what you like best.* And then figure how you can de-calorize it, or substitute a lower calorie something you like just as well, but have perhaps forgotten about eating lately.

Many people make the mistake of trying not to think about food, not fussing about cooking, or food shopping, when watching their weight. On the contrary, you should think more about food, do more cooking, more fussing. You'll need to, because you're going to be inventing new dishes, cooking old dishes in new ways, improvising, thinking more broadly, more creatively about food than you ever have before.

It will astonish you how easy it is to eat what you wish yourself to eat and stay within your calorie program *simply by planning the whole thing out ahead of time*. Your subconscious mind digests the suggestion you plant there by visualizing the next day's eating, and supplies you with the unconscious will and energy to follow your conscious desire.

If circumstances intervene and you don't follow your plan, *don't be annoyed with yourself, or discouraged*. Just continue to plan the next day's eating each night before you go to sleep.

Over a period of time you will find that you follow the pattern you set for yourself. And you're getting the fullest use out of that good head on your shoulders to give yourself what you like to eat and what you want to eat.

Don't rely on invoking that moralistic concept, your "will power." Its invocation tends to arouse various sleeping dogs in your unconscious, described as "won't power." But then you probably have learned that when it comes to changing deep-rooted emotionally based patterns, the "will power" is a very small boy sent on a very big man's errand.

Strategy 3

Eat often. You've heard this before. But do you do it?

Do you have a second breakfast halfway between your first breakfast and lunch? Do you have a late afternoon high tea, or high coffee? Do you have a stomach-warming meal just before you go to bed?

These shouldn't be stand-up nibbles, or cheerless little glasses of sauerkraut juice and a carrot stick. They should be something that's fun to eat. And filling! You should arrange them handsomely on a tray and go sit down in a quiet, pleasant spot. And eat slowly.

Try low-calorie hot chocolate and a plateful of thin cookies—orange or lemon thins, or vanilla wafers or Nabiscos (20 calories each). Or an apple and cheese with waferettes, and coffee. Or a big dish of Sucaryl-sweetened canned fruit, with toasted coconut or "whipped cream" on top, and coffee. Or a bottle of beer with a plateful of hot toasted oysterettes which have been dusted with Parmesan cheese before they went in the oven (1 calorie each).

Use your imagination to please your palate and soothe your savage appetite, so that it has no excuse whatsoever for feeling underprivileged. Naturally, you count the calories in these snacks; add them to your day's total.

If you have been skipping these little time-outs, try resuming them for a few days and see how much they add to the pleasure of life. You'll live longer if you give yourself these respites from the tension and rush of your busy day.

Experience in nutrition laboratories and clinics indicates that with these between-meal meals you want less food at the next meal. Even more important to a continued weight-watching program, they keep your energy and morale high during slump times of the day. Both, as you can see, are essentials to successful weight reduction.

Strategy 4

Eat in style. For women especially, an eye-filling dish also seems to fill the stomach more than a humdrum dish.

If all the meat were taken off a squab and presented to you in a little brown heap, do you think it would be as satisfying to you as when the elegant whole bird is borne in to you, prettily garnished, and you dig each succulent morsel from its delicate hiding place? And don't coffee and toast satisfy you more when you have them from a breakfast tray in bed than when you gulp them standing over the kitchen sink?

When you're limiting your calories you must be especially kind and generous to yourself in every other way you can think of. You must give yourself every eating pleasure you can think of, *except* brute calories unlimited.

Particularly, you must make every dish, every meal, every tray, look as luxurious, as delicious, as beautiful as your ingenuity can devise. This is a vital part of the strategy of making yourself feel pampered, not punished, while you're taking off pounds and taking on youthful vitality.

The fifth "speeder-upper" is so important that it gets a whole section to itself. This is it: EAT MORE SLOWLY.

Strategy 5

To lose faster, eat more slowly. I hope your husband reads this section because this is a formula that men can follow as easily as women. It works on planes or trains, in good restaurants and bad, at home or abroad, whether you're eating alone or in company.

You've heard about eating slowly for digestion's sake. Remember "Fletcherizing"? The big news is that studies now prove conclusively an equally vital connection between how fast we eat and how much we weigh. Eating slowly, by itself, acts *automatically* to reduce the intake of food, and consequently, the patient's weight. It takes time for your stomach to inform your brain that it is content.

There are other rewards about releasing yourself from the bad old habit of gulping food. You enjoy food more when you eat slowly. You taste flavors more. Your teeth and tongue get more fun out of textures. Your nose gets more bang out of aromas. All your senses get in the act—not just your esophagus.

Remember, *haste makes waist*. So put this reminder list where you'll see it often.

Step 1: Concentrate on linger-longer foods—foods that take a lot of eating.

Step 2: Linger longer over your meal—by dividing it in many courses.

Step 3: Distract your attention at mealtime. Remember, the more you talk, the less you eat.

Step 4: Be the last person at the table to finish each course.

Step 5: "Dietize" your food; take much smaller bites, and pause between bites.

Step 6: Check your eating speed (and your improvement) with a clock and a mirror.

THE "BLITZ" DIET: 2 TO 5 POUNDS OFF IN 2 DAYS

People nowadays need short-haul help as well as long-haul help to keep weight down.

I go to visit friends for a long weekend. The food is wonderful. I eat, drink and make merry on a larger scale than at home. And I come home weighing from two to four pounds more.

Maybe it takes you more than a few days to gain that much. But gaining happens to everyone—during holidays, on vacation. During a time of depression or anxiety also, many people tend to eat more, and faster, and oftener. It's a wonderful feeling to be able to shed those few pounds in two days. And you *can*. But you must choose things you love to eat. Because unless you really enjoy what you're eating, you'll find you just don't bother.

If you happen to be fond of cottage cheese you're in luck. . . . Thanks to its unique magic you can take off not less than 2 pounds—and as much as 5 pounds—in *two* days. If you don't, see your doctor. Something's wrong!

The blitz diet

1 cup (8 oz.) cottage cheese, 230 calories; 3 peach halves and juice (I like Diet-Sweet canned Elberta peaches best. Sugarless!), 75 calories; 2 squares of Norwegian flatbread or Ry-Krisp, each brushed

with ¼ teaspoon butter, dusted with ½ teaspoon cinnamon sugar, toasted to a glaze under the broiler. Black coffee or tea. *Total, per meal: 378 calories.* (If you get *no* exercise, or are under 5′5″, *cut* all quantities by ¼; you use less "fuel.") Breakfast, lunch and dinner are the same.

Instead of the dietetic peaches, you may substitute Diet-Sweet apricots (7 halves and juice), or 1 small orange, or ¾ cup fresh berries, or 3 to 4 small stewed prunes in Sucaryl-sweetened syrup. None of these contains more than 75 calories without sugar.

When you would rather have fresh green pepper, tomato, radishes, cucumber, lettuce, crisp rings of Bermuda onion . . . do! You'll lose even faster (fewer calories!).

Like all reducing diets, this has the disadvantage of isolating you from the human herd, especially at dinnertime. But for two days, one can sometimes be odd. If the payoff is big enough, quick enough and *real* enough.

I wrote what you've just finished reading in 1955. (I'm writing THIS in 1977.) *Coronet* magazine picked it (the only diet in the book) to publish. In March 1956. Cottage cheese and peaches. Idiotically simple. But it had *worked.* For me, anyhow. I loved it. Well, it worked for other people, too. They loved it.

Coronet ran another article in September 1956. Title: "The Amazing Blitz Diet and How It Helped Millions Lose 5 Pounds in 2 Days."

"No diet in the past 3 decades ever had so much impact," etc., etc. You get the idea. So. We know all that. Blitz Diet. Everybody discovered cottage cheese. We still eat a lot, the dairy sales figures say. But as a diet, eventually, I got bored with it. As one does with *any* diet.

De-calorizing . . . what this book is about . . . is different. That changes one's outlook; permanently.

Seeing a doctor helps. (Facing the doctor's scale, and possible frown, every week is a big part of that routine.)

And a new quickie diet helps. Whether nutritionists approve or not. Because, in keeping one's weight DOWN, (as in keeping one's morale UP), one needs new stimuli.

Being a try-er, in 21 years, I've tried a lot of slimming combos. Some worked. More didn't. The ones you're going to read now are the ones that worked. They're unscientific, *un*-laboratory tested, unbalanced, and no doubt un-American. And, like the Blitz Diet, they're idiotically simple.

In fact, they aren't diets. (I hate that word, anyhow.) They're just lazy, low calorie food kicks I've loved and lost on.

9 MORE* LAZY LOW CALORIE FOOD KICKS I LOVE AND LOSE ON

With or without pills, when the melons come in, my breakfast changes. So does my weight. I lose winter flab like this:

The 30-30-30 combo
½ cantalope . . . *30 cal.* in its golden, fragrant middle, 1 scant tablespoon of snowy ricotta cheese . . . *30 cal.* A tall glass of iced coffee. 1 crunchy sesame seed stick . . . *30 cal.* Nothing BUT this repeated every few hours for a couple of days leaves me 3 to 5 lbs. lighter. I love it for breakfast all summer.

The Yankee Doodle diet . . . red, white and blue
A mixture of giant blueberries and crisp, sweet, rosy watermelon which has been peeled, cubed and seeded by my twice-a-week cleaning woman. On a big silver platter-full, I plop dollops of creamy ricotta. Coffee. Joy! For 1½ c. watermelon, ¾ c. blueberries, ¼ c. ricotta—only 215 calories, and a lot of ecstatic eating. Add 30 calories for a sesame stick.

Spring's First Fresh Asparagus (S.F.F.A.) splurge
Nothing but the biggest, most sumptuous spears

---

*The blitz diet is the first.

will do the work. Blow the expense! The trick is—
an ORGY. Do NOT buy the spindly, sandy kind.

Buy (and cook) TWICE as much as you think
you could possibly eat. Then you'll have a no-work
salad treat, ready for your next meal. Only 4 or 5
calories in the most colossal spear of S.F.F.A. So I
can eat clean, new SPRING, in its most delectable
form for 200 calories, including lemon juice and 1 T.
melted diet margarine.

I also love: (a) S.F.F.A. with fresh-grated Parmesan (20 cal. per T.); (b) with a sunny fried egg
on top (80 cal.); (c) with frizzles of thin, pink boiled
ham (100 cal. per oz.).

Portable pretzel-apple: office (or on-the-run) lunch

A McIntosh for me (75 cal. each). It's juicy
sweet; tastes so good with the pretzels' crunchy *salt*.
Only 5 calories per thin pretzel stick (like extra-long
kitchen matches). Lots of black coffee.

I keep a tin of pretzel sticks at the office; bring
several apples on Monday. Then (no work, no
thought) a lunch you love is waiting. And it's *filling*.
Why? Because it keeps you biting, chewing, drinking,
eating a long time.

Peppered cucs and c. cheese

A hot-weather special. Slice cucumbers thin, add
onion shavings, salt, lemon juice, a few drops of pepper
sauce, ice cubes. Comes a hunger pang, I can frost a
soup-plate-full with ½ c. Spring-salad-ed cottage cheese
(70 cal.). For crunch, Oysterettes (4 cal. each). With
only 20 calories in a cucumber, even *I* can't eat 50
calories worth at a sitting.

Instant stew: mountainous meal . . . no calories, no work, no thought

Cozy in cold weather, or anytime you feel yawn-
ingly empty. This is for several meals. There's some
ready anytime.

In your stew pan, pour some low calorie Italian
salad dressing. Add 3 fat garlic bulbs put through

your garlic press. Into this rub 1 T. oregano from
between your palms. Brown. Dump into this one 12-
oz. cellophane bag each of frozen chopped onions,
frozen chopped green peppers; one or two 1-lb. cans
of stewed tomatoes; 1 small can Chinese water chestnuts, quartered. Add 1 biggish eggplant,* cut into
inch-square chunks; salt, pepper, Accent.

This needs a good HOTTING, but it doesn't
need *stewing*. I like the fresh-firm texture and taste.

Top your giant plateful with ½ c. Chinese fried
noodles (40 cal.) for extra texture. Or ricotta.

Sausage—plus cozies . . . more mountainous no-calorie meats

1.—Cook ½ head of green cabbage (1 c., 40 cal.)
in salted water with 1 T. lemon juice until crisp-
tender. Just before draining, heat with it 2 quartered
Vienna sausages (39 cal. each) and 1 canned pimiento,
cut in strips.

2.—Treat a head of cauliflower the same way
(3 c. = 90 cal.).

3.—Fresh or canned sauerkraut—all you can eat
—(1 c. = 30 cal.) heated with pennies of Vienna sausage.

Look in your market for variations. For example, Hunter's kraut, complete with caraway seeds. Or
champagned sauerkraut in a jar.

With any one of these, a whooping delicatessen
sesame seed stick, 6″ long, 1½″ wide, only 65
cal.

Salata sorrento . . . red and green and white

Very difficult. Open a chilled can of giant green
asparagus (140 cal. to 15-oz. can). Drain. Dump on
plate. On this, spoon a dozen sweet pickled beet balls.
Top with either ricotta cheese (25 cal. per T.) or
Spring Salad cottage cheese . . . about the same calorie
count. Eat. It's good. It's beautiful.

---

*Or 1 packet frozen cubed zucchini. Or 1 packet Frenched green
beans.

Frutta Italiano ... 100 calories per big sweet serving

Chilled strawberries in thick, sweet syrup (S & W NUTRADIET, red label, and *only 55 calories* in the 8-oz. can). When they're in season, toss in a handful of seedless grapes (1 cal. ea.). Top with a scant ¼ c. yogurt, about 30 cal. With it, coffee and a 30-calorie sesame seed stick.

Now to go back to the book you *started* reading ... written 2 decades ago ... because it's still true ... See next to last paragraph on page vii, lines 19 to 23 on page 1, lines 1 to 5 in paragraph 2 on page 144—oh, well, see the rest of this book all over again.

Quick Calorie Counter

FOOD VALUES IN COMMON PORTIONS AS CALCULATED BY THE U. S. DEPARTMENT OF AGRICULTURE

Data are given in quantities that can be readily adjusted to servings of different sizes. Values for prepared foods and food mixtures have been calculated from typical traditional recipes. Values for cooked vegetables are without added fat.

The following abbreviations are used: gm. for gram; mg. for milligram; I.U. for International Unit; cal. for calories; Tr. for trace. Ounce refers to weight; fluid ounce to measure.

Food and Approximate Measure or Common Weight	Food Energy	Protein	Calcium
MILK AND MILK PRODUCTS:	Cal.	Gm.	Mg.
Buttermilk, from skimmed milk, 1 cup	85	9	288
Milk, cow:			
Fluid, whole, 1 cup	165	9	288
Fluid, nonfat (skimmed), 1 cup	85	9	303
Evaporated (undiluted), 1 cup	345	18	612
Condensed (undiluted), 1 cup	980	25	835
Dry, whole, 1 tablespoon	40	2	76
Dry, nonfat solids, 1 tablespoon	30	3	98

Food and Approximate Measure or Common Weight	Food Energy	Protein	Calcium
MILK AND MILK PRODUCTS—continued	*Cal.*	*Gm.*	*Mg.*
Cheese, 1 ounce:			
Cheddar (1 in. cube)	115	7	206
Cheddar, processed	105	7	191
Cheese foods, Cheddar	90	6	162
Cottage, from skimmed milk	25	6	27
Cream	105	3	19
Swiss	105	8	262
Cream, 1 tablespoon:			
Light	30	Tr.	15
Heavy	50	Tr.	12
Beverages, 1 cup:			
Chocolate (all milk)	240	8	260
Cocoa (all milk)	235	10	298
Chocolate flavored milk	185	8	272
Malted milk	280	12	364
Desserts:			
Blanc mange, 1 cup	275	9	290
Custard, baked, 1 cup	285	13	283
Custard pudding, canned, strained (infant food), 1 ounce	30	1	26
Ice cream, plain:			
1/7 of quart brick	165	3	100
8 fluid ounces	295	6	175
FATS, OILS, RELATED PRODUCTS:			
Bacon, medium fat, broiled or fried, 2 slices	95	4	4
Butter, 1 tablespoon	100	Tr.	3
Fats, cooking (vegetable fats):			
1 cup	1770	0	0
1 tablespoon	110	0	0
Lard, 1 tablespoon	125	0	0
Margarine, 1 tablespoon	100	Tr.	3
Oils, salad or cooking, 1 tablespoon	125	0	0

Food and Approximate Measure or Common Weight	Food Energy	Protein	Calcium

FATS, OILS, RELATED PRODUCTS—continued	Cal.	Gm.	Mg.
Salad dressings, 1 tablespoon:			
French	60	Tr.	0
Home-cooked	30	1	15
Mayonnaise	90	Tr.	2

EGGS:			
Eggs, raw, medium:			
1 whole	75	6	26
1 white	15	3	2
1 yolk	60	3	25
Eggs, dried, whole, 1 cup	640	51	205

MEAT, POULTRY, FISH:			
Beef, 3 ounces, without bone, cooked:			
Chuck	265	2	9
Hamburger	315	19	8
Sirloin	255	20	9
Beef, canned:			
Corned beef, medium fat, 3 ounces	180	22	17
Corned beef hash, 3 ounces	120	12	22
Strained (infant food), 1 ounce	30	5	3
Beef, dried, 2 ounces	115	19	11
Beef and vegetable stew, 1 cup	250	13	31
Chicken, canned, boned, 3 ounces	170	25	12
Chili con carne, canned (without beans), ⅓ cup	170	9	32
Clams, raw, meat only, 4 ounces	90	15	109
Cod, dried, 1 ounce	105	23	14
Crab meat, canned or cooked, 3 ounces	90	14	38
Flounder, raw, 4 ounces	80	17	69
Haddock, fried, 1 fillet (4 by 3 by ½ in.)	160	19	18
Halibut, broiled, 1 steak (4 by 3 by ½ in.)	230	33	18
Heart, beef, raw, 3 ounces	90	14	8
Kidneys, beef, raw, 3 ounces	120	13	8

Food and Approximate Measure or Common Weight	Food Energy	Protein	Calcium
MEAT, POULTRY, FISH— continued	*Cal.*	*Gm.*	*Mg.*
Lamb, leg roast, cooked, 3 ounces	230	20	9
Lamb, canned, strained (infant food), 1 ounce	30	4	5
Liver, beef, fried, 2 ounces	120	13	5
Liver, canned, strained (infant food), 1 ounce	30	5	7
Mackerel, canned, solids and liquid, 3 ounces	155	16	157
Oysters, meat only, raw, 1 cup (13–19 medium size oysters, selects)	200	24	226
Oyster stew, 1 cup with 6 to 8 oysters	245	17	262
Pork loin or chops, cooked, 3 ounces without bone	285	20	9
Pork, cured ham, cooked, 3 ounces without bone	340	20	9
Pork luncheon meat, canned, spiced, 2 ounces	165	8	5
Salmon, canned, pink, 3 ounces	120	17	159
Sardines, canned in oil, drained solids, 3 ounces	180	22	328
Sausage:			
Bologna, 1 piece (1 by 1½ in diam.)	465	31	19
Frankfurter, 1 cooked	125	7	3
Pork, bulk, canned, 4 ounces	340	17	10
Scallops, raw, 4 ounces	90	17	29
Shad, raw, 4 ounces	190	21	—
Shrimp, canned, meat only, 3 ounces	110	23	98
Soups, canned, ready-to-serve:			
Beef, 1 cup	100	6	15
Chicken, 1 cup	75	4	20
Chicken, strained (infant food), 1 ounce	15	1	11
Clam chowder, 1 cup	85	5	36
Tongue, beef, raw, 4 ounces	235	19	10

Food and Approximate Measure or Common Weight	Food Energy	Protein	Calcium
MEAT, POULTRY, FISH— continued	Cal.	Gm.	Mg.
Tuna fish, drained solids, 3 ounces	170	25	7
Veal cutlet, cooked, 3 ounces without bone	185	24	10
MATURE BEANS AND PEAS; NUTS:			
Almonds, shelled, unblanched, 1 cup	850	26	361
Beans, canned or cooked, 1 cup:			
Red kidney	230	15	102
Navy or other varieties with:			
Pork and tomato sauce	295	15	107
Pork and molasses	325	15	146
Beans, lima, dry, 1 cup	610	38	124
Brazil nuts, shelled, 1 cup	905	20	260
Coconut, dried, shredded (sweetened), 1 cup	345	2	27
Cowpeas, dry, 1 cup	685	46	154
Peanuts, roasted, shelled, 1 cup	805	39	107
Peanut butter, 1 tablespoon	90	4	12
Peas, split, dry, 1 cup	690	49	66
Pecans, 1 cup halves	750	10	80
Soybeans, dry, 1 cup	695	73	477
Walnuts, English, 1 cup halves	655	15	83
VEGETABLES:			
Asparagus:			
Cooked, 1 cup spears	35	4	33
Canned, green, 6 spears, medium size	20	2	18
Canned, bleached, 6 spears, medium size	20	2	15
Beans, lima, immature, cooked, 1 cup	150	8	46
Beans, snap, green, cooked, 1 cup	25	2	45
Beets, cooked, diced, 1 cup	70	2	35
Broccoli, cooked, flower stalks, 1 cup	45	5	195

Food and Approximate Measure or Common Weight	Food Energy	Protein	Calcium
VEGETABLES—continued	Cal.	Gm.	Mg.
Brussels sprouts, cooked, 1 cup	60	6	44
Cabbage, 1 cup:			
Raw, shredded	25	1	46
Cooked	40	2	78
Carrots:			
Raw, grated, 1 cup	45	1	43
Cooked, diced, 1 cup	45	1	38
Canned, strained (infant food), 1 oz.	10	Tr.	7
Cauliflower, cooked, flower buds, 1 cup	30	3	26
Celery, 1 cup:			
Raw, diced	20	1	50
Cooked, diced	25	2	65
Collards, cooked, 1 cup	75	7	473
Corn, sweet:			
Cooked, 1 ear (5 in. long)	85	3	5
Canned, solids and liquid, 1 cup	170	5	10
Cowpeas, immature seed, cooked, 1 cup	150	11	59
Cucumbers, raw, 6 slices (⅛ in. thick, center section)	5	Tr.	5
Dandelion greens, cooked, 1 cup	80	5	337
Endive, raw, 1 pound	90	7	359
Kale, cooked, 1 cup	45	4	248
Lettuce, headed, raw, 2 large or 4 small leaves	5	1	11
Mushrooms, canned, solids and liquid, 1 cup	30	3	17
Mustard greens, cooked, 1 cup	30	3	308
Okra, cooked, 8 pods (3 in. long, ⅝ in. diam.)	30	2	70
Onions, raw:			
Mature, 1 onion (2½ in. diam.)	50	2	35
Young green, 6 small onions without tops	25	Tr.	68
Parsnips, cooked, 1 cup	95	2	88

Food and Approximate Measure or Common Weight	Food Energy	Protein	Calcium
VEGETABLES—continued	Cal.	Gm.	Mg.
Peas, green:			
Cooked, 1 cup	110	8	35
Canned, strained (infant food), 1 ounce	15	1	5
Peppers, green, raw, 1 medium	15	1	7
Potatoes:			
Baked, 1 medium (2½ in. diam.)	95	2	13
Boiled in skin, 1 medium (2½ in. diam.)	120	3	16
Boiled after peeling, 1 medium (2½ in. diam.)	105	3	14
French-fried, 8 pieces (2 by ½ by ½ in.)	155	2	12
Potato chips, 10 medium (2 in. diam.)	110	1	6
Pumpkin, canned, 1 cup	75	2	46
Radishes, raw, 4 small	5	Tr.	7
Rutabagas, cooked, cubed or sliced, 1 cup	50	1	85
Sauerkraut, canned, drained solids, 1 cup	30	2	54
Soybean sprouts, raw 1 cup	50	7	51
Spinach:			
Cooked, 1 cup	45	6	223
Canned. strained (infant food), 1 ounce	5	1	22
Squash:			
Summer, cooked, diced, 1 cup	35	1	32
Winter, baked, mashed, 1 cup	95	4	49
Winter, canned, strained (infant food), 1 ounce	10	Tr.	9
Sweet potatoes, peeled, 1 sweet potato:			
Baked (5 by 2 in.)	185	3	44
Boiled (5 by 2½ in.)	250	4	62
Tomatoes:			
Raw, 1 medium (by 2½ in.)	30	2	16
Canned or cooked, 1 cup	45	2	27

Food and Approximate Measure or Common Weight	Food Energy	Protein	Calcium
VEGETABLES—continued	Cal.	Gm.	Mg.
Tomato juice, canned, 1 cup	50	2	17
Turnips, cooked, diced, 1 cup	40	1	62
Turnips, cooked, 1 cup	45	4	376
Vegetables, mixed, canned, strained (infant food), 1 ounce	10	Tr.	9
FRUITS:			
Apples, raw, 1 medium (2½ in. diam.)	75	Tr.	8
Apple juice, fresh or canned, 1 cup	125	Tr.	15
Apple betty, 1 cup	345	4	35
Applesauce, canned, sweetened, 1 cup	185	1	10
Apricots:			
Raw, 3 apricots	55	1	17
Canned in syrup, 4 medium halves and 2 tablespoons syrup	95	1	12
Canned, strained (infant food), 1 ounce	15	Tr.	6
Dried, cooked, unsweetened, fruit and liquid, 1 cup	240	5	80
Avocados, raw, ½ peeled fruit (3½ by 3¼ in.)	280	2	11
Bananas, raw, 1 medium (6 by 1½ in.)	90	1	8
Blackberries, raw, 1 cup	80	2	46
Blueberries, raw, 1 cup	85	1	22
Cantaloupes, raw, ½ melon (5 in. diam.)	35	1	31
Cherries, 1 cup, pitted:			
Raw	65	1	19
Canned, red, sour	120	2	28
Cranberry sauce, sweetened, 1 cup	550	Tr.	22
Dates, "fresh" and dried, pitted and cut, 1 cup	505	4	128
Figs, raw, 3 small (1½ in. diam.)	90	2	62

Food and Approximate Measure or Common Weight	Food Energy	Protein	Calcium
FRUITS—continued	Cal.	Gm.	Mg.
Figs, dried, 1 large (2 by 1 in.)	55	1	39
Fruit cocktail, canned, solids and liquid, 1 cup	180	1	23
Grapefruit, raw, 1 cup sections	75	1	43
Grapefruit juice:			
Canned, unsweetened, 1 cup	90	1	20
Frozen concentrate, 6-ounce can	295	4	63
Grapes, 1 cup:			
American type (slip skin)	85	2	20
European type (adherent skin)	100	1	26
Grape juice, bottled, 1 cup	170	1	25
Lemon juice, fresh, 1 cup	60	1	34
Lime juice, fresh, 1 cup	60	1	34
Oranges, 1 medium (3 in. diam.)	70	1	51
Orange juice:			
Fresh, 1 cup	110	2	47
Canned, unsweetened, 1 cup	110	2	25
Frozen, concentrate, 6-ounce can	300	5	69
Papayas raw, cubed, 1 cup	70	1	36
Peaches:			
Raw, 1 medium (2½ by 2 in. diam.)	45	1	8
Canned in syrup, solids and liquid, 1 cup	175	1	13
Canned, strained (infant food), 1 ounce	15	Tr.	2
Dried, cooked, unsweetened, 1 cup (10–12 halves and 6 tablespoons liquid)	225	2	38
Pears:			
Raw, 1 pear (3 by 2½ in. diam.)	95	1	20
Canned in syrup, 2 medium size halves and 2 tablespoons syrup	80	Tr.	9
Canned, strained (infant food), 1 ounce	15	Tr.	3

Food and Approximate Measure or Common Weight	Food Energy	Protein	Calcium
FRUITS—continued	Cal.	Gm.	Mg.
Persimmons, Japanese, raw, seedless kind, 1 persimmon (2¼ in. diam.)	95	1	7
Pineapple:			
Raw, diced, 1 cup	75	1	22
Canned in syrup, 2 small or 1 large slice and 2 tablespoons juice	95	Tr.	35
Pineapple juice, canned, 1 cup	120	1	37
Plums, raw, 1 plum (2 in. diam.)	30	Tr.	10
Prunes, cooked, unsweetened, 1 cup (16–18 prunes and ⅓ cup liquid)	310	3	62
Prune juice, canned, 1 cup	170	1	60
Raisins, dried, 1 cup	430	4	125
Raspberries, red, raw, 1 cup	70	1	49
Rhubarb, cooked with sugar, 1 cup	385	1	*112
Strawberries:			
Raw, 1 cup	55	1	42
Frozen, 3 ounces	90	1	19
Tangerines, 1 medium (2½ in. diam.)	35	1	27
Tangerine juice, canned, 1 cup	95	2	47
Watermelons, ½ slice (¾ by 10 in.)	45	1	11
GRAIN PRODUCTS:			
Barley, pearled, light, dry, 1 cup	710	17	32
Biscuits, baking powder, enriched flour, 1 biscuit (2½ in. diam.)	130	3	83
Bran flakes, 1 cup	115	4	24

*Calcium may not be usable because of presence of oxalic acid.

Food and Approximate Measure or Common Weight	Food Energy	Protein	Calcium
GRAIN PRODUCTS—continued	Cal.	Gm.	Mg.
Breads, 1 slice:			
Boston brown, unenriched	105	2	89
Rye	55	2	17
White, unenriched, 4 per cent nonfat milk solids	65	2	18
White, enriched, 4 per cent nonfat milk solids	65	2	18
White, enriched, 6 per cent nonfat milk solids	65	2	21
Whole wheat	55	2	22
Cakes:			
Angel food, 2-in sector (1/12 of cake, 8 in. diam.)	110	3	2
Doughnuts, cake-type, 1 doughnut	135	2	23
Foundation, 1 square (3 by 2 by 1¾ in.)	230	4	82
Foundation, plain icing, 2-in sector, layer cake (1/16 of cake, 10 in. diam.)	410	6	121
Fruit cake, dark, 1 piece (2 by 2 by ½ in.)	105	2	29
Gingerbread, 1 piece (2 by 2 by 2 in.)	180	2	63
Plain cake and cupcakes, 1 cupcake (2¾ in. diam.)	130	3	62
Sponge, 2-in. sector (1/12 of cake, 8 in. diam.)	115	3	11
Cereal foods, dry, precooked (infant food), 1 ounce	105	4	185
Cookies, plain and assorted, 1 3-inch cookie	110	2	6
Corn bread or muffins made with enriched, degermed corn meal, 1 muffin (2¾ in. diam.)	105	3	67
Corn flakes, 1 cup	95	2	3
Corn grits, degermed, cooked, 1 cup:			
Unenriched	120	3	2
Enriched	120	3	2

Food and Approximate Measure or Common Weight	Food Energy	Protein	Calcium
GRAIN PRODUCTS—continued	*Cal.*	*Gm.*	*Mg.*
Crackers:			
Graham, 4 small or 2 medium	55	1	3
Soda, plain, 2 crackers			
(2½ in. diam.)	45	1	2
Farina, enriched, cooked, 1 cup	105	3	7
Macaroni, cooked, 1 cup:			
Unenriched	210	7	13
Enriched	210	7	13
Muffins, made with enriched			
flour, 1 muffin			
(2¾ in. diam.)	135	4	99
Noodles, containing egg,			
unenriched, cooked, 1 cup	105	4	6
Oatmeal or rolled oats:			
Cooked, 1 cup	150	5	21
Precooked (infant food),			
dry, 1 oz.	105	4	225
Pancakes, baked wheat, with			
enriched flour, 1 cake			
(4-in. diam.)	60	2	43
Pies, 4-inch sector (9 in. diam.):			
Apple	330	3	9
Custard	265	7	162
Lemon meringue	300	4	24
Mince	340	3	22
Pumpkin	265	5	70
Pretzels, 5 small sticks	20	Tr.	1
Rice, cooked, 1 cup:			
Converted	205	4	14
White or milled	200	4	13
Rice, puffed, 1 cup	55	1	3
Rolls, plain, enriched, 1 roll			
(12 per pound)	120	3	21
Spaghetti, unenriched, cooked,			
1 cup	220	7	13
Waffles, baked, with enriched			
flour, 1 waffle (4½ by			
5⅝ by ½ in.)	215	7	144

Food and Approximate Measure or Common Weight	Food Energy	Protein	Calcium
GRAIN PRODUCTS—continued	Cal.	Gm.	Mg.
Wheat flours:			
Whole, 1 cup stirred	400	16	49
All purpose or family flour:			
Unenriched, 1 cup sifted	400	12	18
Enriched, 1 cup sifted	400	12	18
Wheat germ, 1 cup stirred	245	17	57
Wheat, shredded, 1 large			
biscuit, 1 oz.	100	3	13
SUGARS, SWEETS:			
Candy, 1 ounce:			
Caramels	120	1	36
Chocolate, sweetened, milk	145	2	61
Fudge, plain	115	Tr.	14
Hard	110	0	0
Marshmallows	90	1	0
Chocolate syrup, 1 tablespoon	40	Tr.	3
Honey, strained or extracted,			
1 tablespoon	60	Tr.	1
Jams, marmalades, preserves,			
1 tablespoon	55	Tr.	2
Molasses, cane, 1 tablespoon:			
Light	50	0	33
Blackstrap	45	0	116
Syrup, table blends, 1 tablespoon	55	0	9
Sugar, 1 tablespoon:			
Granulated, cane or beet	50	0	0
Brown	50	0	0
MISCELLANEOUS:			
Beverages, carbonated, kola			
type, 1 cup	105	0	0
Bouillon cubes, 1 cube	2	Tr.	0
Chocolate, unsweetened, 1 ounce	140	2	28
Gelatin dessert, plain, ready-to-			
serve, 1 cup	155	4	0
Olives, pickled "mammoth" size,			
10 olives:			
Green	70	1	48
Ripe, Mission variety	105	1	48

Food and Approximate Measure or Common Weight	Food Energy	Protein	Calcium
MISCELLANEOUS—continued	*Cal.*	*Gm.*	*Mg.*
Pickles:			
Dill, cucumber, 1 large (4 in. long)	15	1	34
Sweet, cucumber or mixed, 1 pickle (2¾ in. long)	20	Tr.	3
Sherbet, ½ cup	120	1	48
Vinegar, 1 tablespoon	2	0	1
White sauce, medium, 1 cup	430	11	305
Yeast:			
Compressed, baker's, 1 ounce	25	3	8
Dried brewer's, 1 tablespoon	20	3	8

Index

Alcoholic beverages, 135–144
  beer, 139–143
  calories per ounce, 136
  highballs, 137
  wine spritzers, 138
Almonds (filet of sole), 6
Angel food cake mix, 25–27
  cookies, 28
  upside-down cakes, 27
    nutted apricot, 27
    pineapple chunk, 27–28
Appetizers, 36, 69–72
  clams, 71–72
  cocktail cheese sticks, 23
Apple pie, 24–25
Apricots, nutted apricot upside-down cake, 27
Artichokes, 95
Asparagus, with hollandaise sauce, 104
Au gratin vegetables, cream sauce for, 15

Bacon, 122
Bananas, 30, 114
Béarnaise sauce, 22
Beef: chili con carne, 82; chipped, 15, 55; corned beef and cabbage, 86; dried, 55; goulash, 84; gravy, 105; pot roast, 82; roast beef hash, 87–88; sauce with boiled, 102; Stroganoff, 84
Beer, 139–143
Beverages: alcoholic, 135–144; beer, 139–143; coffee, 67–68; de-calorized, 42–43, 64–68; fruit juices, 42; hot chocolate, 43; lemonade, 67; Mexican chocolate, 68; milk shakes, 68; non-fat dry milk, 42–43; sugarless soft drinks, 24, 25, 31, 43, 65, 67
Blender recipes, 126
  canapé spread, basic, 70–71
  frosting, basic, 31
    (chocolate; maple)
  hollandaise, 21–22
    (dill; mint; chive; Béarnaise Sauce)
  milk shakes, 68
    (chocolate; peach;

Blender recipes (*cont.*)
    strawberry; apricot; pineapple; raspberry; banana)
  potatoes, aerated, 96
Blitz diet, 164–166
Blueberries, 19, 24
Borsch soup, 5
Brandy, used in cooking, 5
Bread, low-calorie, 36
Brewer's yeast, 55
Broccoli, hollandaise sauce, 104
Brownies, nutty, 28
Butter, whipped, 19, 61
Butterscotch sauce, 32

Cabbage, corned beef and, 86
Cakes
  angel food cake mix, 25–26
    cookies, 28
    upside-down cakes, 27
  cake mixes
    angel food, 25–26
    gingerbread, 29
  chocolate angel cake, 27
  chocolate chip angel cake, 27
  coconut balls, 28
  gingerbread mix, 29
  ice cream, 28
  marble, 27
  pineapple upside-down, 27–28
  sunshine sponge, 26–27
  twentieth-century master recipe, 25
  upside-down, 27

  nutted apricot, 27
  pineapple chunk, 27–28
Calorie counters, 34, 120, 159, 170–183
Canapés, 69–72
Candies, de-calorized, 41
Casseroles, 13–17, 84, 85, 88–89
Celery, canapés, 71
Cheese: cocktail cheese sticks, 23; cottage, 54–55; cheesecake, 114–115; curry "cream" cheese spread, 72; de-calorized hollandaise sauce, 21–22; mixed with dehydrated onion soup, 5; peppers stuffed with, 94; roquefort spread, 72; salads, 59–60, 164–165; sandwich fillings, 60; served with fruit, 60; "sour cream," 95; used for whipped cream, 11
cottage, 59
  as substitute for flour, 8–9
  canapés, 70
  de-calorized pastry, 22–23
  ginger drop cookies, 30
farmer, 60–61
  for canapés, 70
macaroni and, 90
parmesan, 5–6
roquefort spread, 72
sauces, 16
soufflé, 16–17

Cheesecake, 15-minute de-calorized, 114–115
Cherries, *flambé*, 5
Chewing gums, de-calorized, 43
Chicken: à la king, 15; breasts, 55; chow mein, 83; curry, 16; fried or in-a-basket, 88–89
Chili con carne, 82
Chipped beef, 15, 55
Chocolate: cake, 27; frostings, 31–32; de-calorized sauce, 35–36, 44; hot, 43; Mexican, 68; nutty brownies, 28; sugarless syrups, 35–36, 44
Chow mein, 83
Clams, 69, 71–72, 101
Cocktail sauces, 102, 103
Coffee, 67–68
    frosted, 67–68
Cookies: date-nut bars, 28; de-calorized pastry, 23; ginger drop, 30; low-calorie, 35, 41–42; nutty brownies, 28; rolled ginger, 30–31
Corn
    muffins, 19
    sweet corn pudding, 94–95
Corned beef and cabbage, 86
Cottage cheese, whipped, 70
Crab meat, 15, 16
Cranberry sauce, 10, 106–107

Cream
    sauces, 13–17
        3-minute de-fatted, 14
    made from cottage cheese, 11
    whipped, substitutes, 6, 11
Creole sauce, 100–101
Cucumbers, canapés, 71
Curried dishes, cream sauce, 16

Date-nut bars, 28
Desserts, 36–42, 108–116
    banana *flambé* kirsch, 114
    cheesecake, 114–115
    de-calorized, 36–42
    gelatin, 39–40
        plum ring, 113
    green grape compote, 114
    ice cream, 108–113
        de-calorized, 112–113
    lemon meringue pie, 116
    list of low-calorie fruits, 116
    pastry; *see* Pastry
    zabaione or zabaglione, 114
Diets, 48–49; two-day, 164–166
Duck, à l'orange, 85

Eggs, 124
    curried, 16
    whites
        as a substitute for flour, 8–9
        de-fatted muffins, 18–20
        whipped cream, 6

Eggs (*cont.*)
yolks for zabaglione, 114

Fish, 75–76
cream sauces for, 14–15; creole sauce, 100–101; filet of sole amandine, 6; lemon cocktail sauce, 101–103; planked, 123; scalloped, 15; shellfish, 76
Flavoring extracts, 107–108
Flour, 8–9, 46, 55
Frankfurters, as a garnish for soups, 72
French dressings, de-calorized, 45, 104–105
for moistening canapé spreads, 70
Frostings and fillings, de-calorized: banana cream, 30; butterscotch, 32; chocolate, 31–32; lemon, 31; lemon cream, 31; pineapple cream, 29; whipped cream filling or topping, 26, 31
Fruits: banana *flambé* kirsch, 114; as a first course, 77–78; frozen, 116; gelatin fall fruit soufflé, 40; gelatin plum ring, 113; glazes, 115; green grape compote, 114; juices, 42; list of low-calorie, 35–36, 37, 38, 116;

sherbet, 110; syrups, sugarless, 44

Garnishes, 38–39, 73–74, 113
Gelatin desserts, 39–40
cheesecake, 114–115
fall fruit soufflé salad, 40
plum ring, 113
Gingerbread mix, 29–30
Glazes, fruit, 115
Goulash, 84
Grapes, green, compote, 114
Gravies, 105–106

Hollandaise sauce, de-calorized recipe, 21–22, 104
Honey-butter, 19

Ice cream, 108–113

Jams and jellies
sucaryl-sweetened, 19, 44–45

Lamb, 22, 79
Leftover meats and fowl, 79
Lemon: meringue pie, 116; sugarless cake filling, 31–32
Lemonade, 67
Liqueurs, served on fruit, 5
Lobster, 15, 16

Macaroni, with cheese, 90
Maple: sugarless syrup, 20–21, 43–44

Mayonnaise, low-calorie, 35, 45
  sauces made with, 102–103
Meats, 78–89
  beef Stroganoff, 84; broiling, 79; chili con carne, 82; chipped beef, 15, 55; chow mein, 83; corned beef and cabbage, 86; defatting, 7–8, 78–79; duck à l'orange, 85; fried chicken, 88–89; frying, 79; goulash, 84; hamburg, 8; veal stew, 87; pot roast, 82–83; roast beef hash, 87–88; spaghetti with meat sauce, 91; utilizing leftovers, 79; veal scallopini, 86
Milk
  dry skimmed, 42–43, 54, 66
    whipped cream, 11
  evaporated
    banana cream filling, 30
    pineapple cream filling, 29
    whipped cream, 11
  nonfat dry, 42–43, 56, 66
  shakes, 68
  skimmed, 54, 56
    puddings made with, 38
Muffins, recipe for defatted, 9, 18–19; blueberry, 19; corn, 19; date, 19; nut, 19; raisin, 19; traditional recipe, 18
Mushrooms, 95
  à la king dishes, 15–16
  canapé bases, 71
  sautéed with "sour cream," 95

Newburg sauce, 16
Noodles, 89–91
  fried, 83
Nuts
  black walnuts on boiled onions, 94
  date-nut bars, 28
  muffins, 19

Onions, 5, 11, 71
Orange, 85

Pancakes, puff, 20–21
Pastry, 22–23; apple pie, 24–25; blueberry pie, 24; cocktail cheese sticks, 23; de-calorized pie crust, 22–23; lemon meringue pie, 116; pumpkin pie, 24
Peaches, and cottage cheese salad, 164–165
Peanut butter, 46
Peppers, cheese stuffed, 94
Pineapple, 27–28, 29
Plum ring, 113
Pork: low calorie content of, 79; chow mein, 83; roasting, 80
Pot roast, 82–83
Potatoes, 15, 96

Protein, 48–52
Puddings, de-calorized, 38
  sweet corn, 94–95
Pumpkin pie, 24

Raisin muffins, 19
Rice, wild, 87
Russian dressing, 103

Saccharin, 46
Salads, 76–78, 91–92
  as a first course, 72–73
  chilled cream, 101–102
  de-calorized dressings,
    45
  fall fruit soufflé, 40
  French dressings, 45,
    104–105
  mayonnaise, 5, 35, 45,
    102–103
  peach and cottage
    cheese, 164–165
  potato, 96
Salmon, 47, 102
Sandwich fillings, 59
Sauces, 97–108; à la king,
  15–16; au gratin, 15;
  barbecue, 103; Béar-
  naise, 22; brown,
  105–106; butter-
  scotch, 32; cheese,
  16; chilled cream
  dressing, 101; clam-
  tomato, 101; cocktail,
  102; cranberry, 10,
  106–107; cream, 13–
  17, 99; creole, 100–
  101; curry, 16; gra-
  vies, 105–106; hollan-
  daise, 5, 104 (de-cal-
  orized, 21–22); horse-
  radish, 102; meat for

spaghetti, 91; mush-
  room, 99; mustard,
  103; Newburg, 16;
  Russian dressing, 103;
  for scalloped dishes,
  15; Spanish, 100–
  101; tomato, 100–
  101; white, 3-minute
  defatted, 14
Sherry, used in cooking,
  16, 74
Shrimps, 16, 83, 100–101
Soft drinks, de-calorized,
  carbonated, 43
Sorbitol, 38
Soufflés: fall fruit, 40;
  low-calorie cheese,
  16–17
Soups, 5, 72–75
Sour cream, made from
  cottage cheese, 95
Spaghetti: with meat
  sauce, 89–91
Squash, pseudo-sweet po-
  tato pluff, 93–94
Stew, veal, 87
Sucaryl (sodium cycla-
  mate), 9–10, 37, 45–
  46
Syrups, de-calorized, 43–
  45; chocolate, 44;
  fruit, 44; maple, 43–
  44

Tomatoes, 5, 69, 99–101
Tuna fish, 47, 83, 89
Veal, 15, 84, 86, 87
Vegetables, 15, 91–96

Waffles, de-calorized, 20
Wheat germ, 54

Whipped cream substitutes, 6, 11
White sauce, 14, 16–17
Wine, in cooking, 5, 114, 138

Yeast, 54–55
Yogurt, 101
Yogurt basic cream dressing: sauces, 101
Zabaglione, 114

Facts at Your Fingertips!